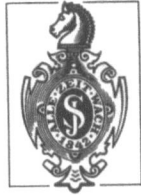

F. S. Weill   A. Le Mouël

Exercises in Diagnostic Ultrasonography of the Abdomen

Translated by R. Chambers

With 361 Figures

Springer-Verlag
Berlin Heidelberg New York Tokyo 1983

FRANCIS S. WEILL, M.D.
Professor of Radiology, University of Besançon, Head Department
of Radiology, University Hospital, 2, Place Saint-Jacques,
F-25000 Besançon

ARLETTE LE MOUËL, M.D.
Senior Radiologist, Head Department of Radiology, University Hospital,
2, Place Saint-Jacques, F-25000 Besançon

Translator:
RICHARD CHAMBERS, 9 bis rue de la Grette, F-25000 Besançon

Title of the original French edition:
Exercices de diagnostic abdominal by F. S. Weill, A. Le Mouël
© Editions Vigot Freres, Paris, 1982

ISBN-13: 978-3-540-12228-9   e-ISBN-13: 978-3-642-68986-4
DOI: 10.1007/978-3-642-68986-4

Library of Congress Cataloging in Publication Data. Weill, Francis Samuel, 1933- Exercises
in diagnostic ultrasonography of the abdomen. Translation of: Exercices de diagnostic
abdominal. 1. Abdomen–Radiography–Problems, exercises, etc. 2. Diagnosis, Ultrasonic-
Problems, exercises, etc. I. Le Mouël, A. (Arlette) II. Title. RC944.W3813 1983 617'.5507543
83-4658

2121/3130-543210

Contents

Introduction

This book of diagnostic exercises cannot be used to good advantage without a good grasp of elementary sonoanatomy and the most common pathologic images[1]. We have tried to follow a pedagogical progression from the simple to the complicated for each group of clinical situations. We recommend that the sonograms at the beginning of each case study be thoroughly analysed before proceeding to the commentaries which explain the grounds for the final diagnosis. These explanatory remarks are accompanied by the same sonograms, but with arrows and letters added so as to pinpoint the details referred to as the diagnosis progresses. In reading the commentaries it will therefore be a good idea to cover over the figures in which the details are picked out for you, uncovering them one by one as required.

---

1 Which the reader may obtain from our previous books:
  Ultrasonography of Digestive Diseases (Mosby Publ., 2nd Ed., 1982)
  Renal Sonography (Springer Verlag, 1981)

Chapter 1

In Which the Reader is Invited to Clean His Glasses

1.1. Mrs. Beech, 75 years, has the complexion of a young girl, but she is losing weight and complains of epigastric pain. She has undergone a whole series of conventional radiological procedures; this may be good news for the film manufacturers, but it has not aided in the diagnosis. Finally, she is referred for an ultrasound examination.

Look first at ultrasonic cuts 1.1a, b (transverse), then 1.1d (sagittal).

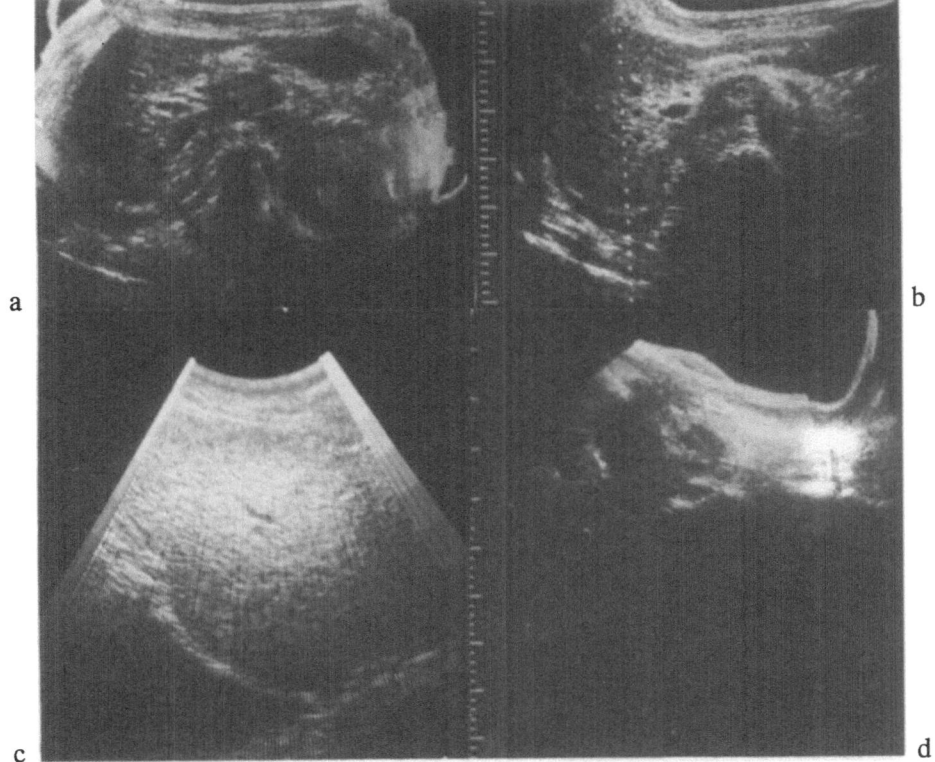

a   b

c   d

Fig. 1.1

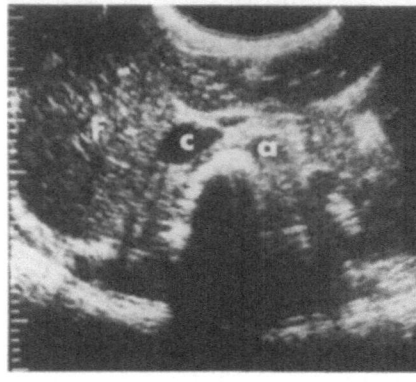

Fig. 1.1e

There is a large abnormality here. If you haven't discovered it, it will become obvious if you compare these pathologic images with the normal image in Fig. 1.1e, which is from another individual.

What is this abnormality?

It is clearly a deep sonolucent mass, with smooth limits and a small central echogenic zone (↓ below).

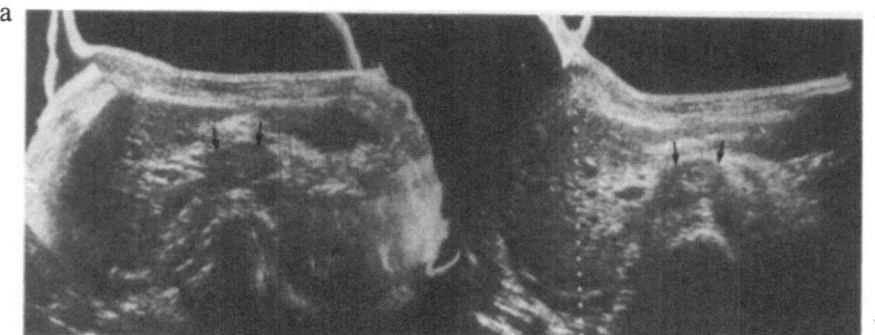

Fig. 1.1

The mass is also seen in sagittal section (↓ Fig. 1.1d, below)

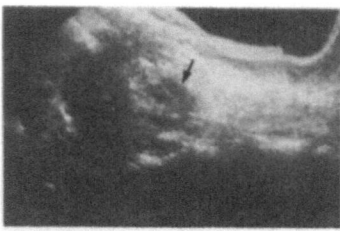

Fig. 1.1d

4

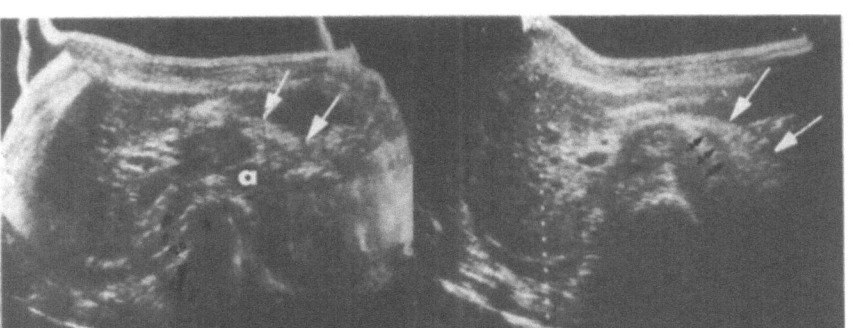

Fig. 1.1

What is its relationship to the pancreas?

The comma shaped reflective echotexture (↓) of the latter is well marked (see above, Fig. 1.1a, b). It is underlined along its posterior aspect by the transparency of the splenic vein (↕ Fig. 1.1b).

In this case, we are confronted with a mass located anterior to the large vessels (*a* = aorta) and within the posterior part of the pancreatic head. It forces part of the pancreatic tissue forward.
Before we continue our discussion of the nature of this mass, carefully study Fig. 1.1a (above). As good internists we now want to know the condition of a particular anatomic structure. What should we assess?

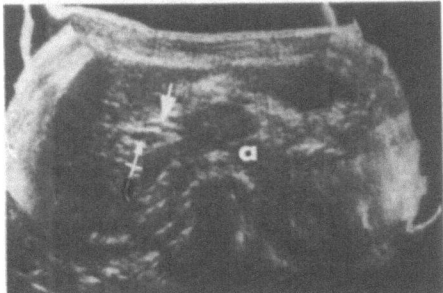

Fig. 1.1a

We assess the common bile duct and find the beginning of a "gun sign" (white arrow and crossed arrow above). The diameter of the bile duct (white arrow), anterior to the portal vein (↑), is half the diameter of the latter. This is the upper normal limit for the relationship between these two diameters. Most likely, Mrs. Beech will soon be losing her young girl's complexion in exchange for one more Asiatic in appearance.

5

Now, carefully study Fig. 1.1b below. You have thirty seconds to try to extend the list of Mrs. Beech's problems. You note...

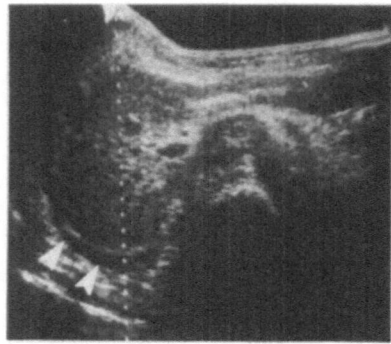

Fig. 1.1b

...You note, posterior to the liver, a sonotransparent, comma-shaped fluid collection (white arrowheads).

It corresponds to?...

...to a pleural effusion. A small ascitic strip would be in an anterior or lateral position in relation to the liver. This image is also visible in Fig. 1.1a below (arrowheads).

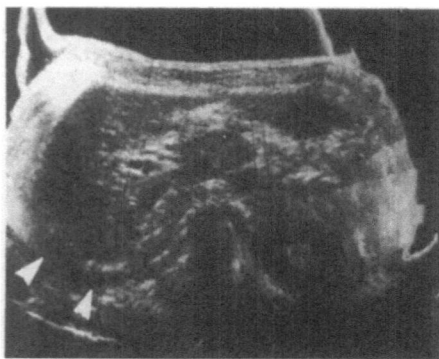

Fig. 1.1a

If you're not convinced look at Fig. 1.1c (p. 3, then next page).

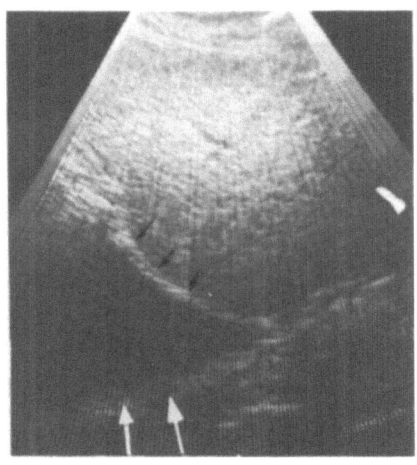

Fig. 1.1c

The figure is a sagittal section of the right upper quadrant. It disctinctly shows a fluid collection above the diaphragm (black arrows). Due to this liquid contrast, the posterior thoracic wall is visualized (white arrows). Normally, no echo appears above the dome of the liver and the diaphragm.

A puncture will show that this effusion is hemorrhagic.

For the moment we can conclude that there is a mass of the *cephalic pancreatic region,* which is beginning to *compress the common bile duct* and is accompanied by a *hemorrhagic pleural effusion,* most likely metastatic.

Logically, this image of a retroperitoneal mass should be caused by an adenopathy, since it forces the splenic vein as well as the pancreatic tissue forward. Can a pancreatic carcinoma cause the same type of anterior bulging? It seems improbable since the branches of the portal system are retropancreatic: logically they should be forced backward. In fact, pancreatic tumors as they progress deeper usually do compress these portal branches posteriorly. However, when the tumor develops in the uncinate process, which is posterior to the mesenteric vein, then like an adenopathy it forces the pancreas forward (see also Fig. 1.1f–h, below).

fig 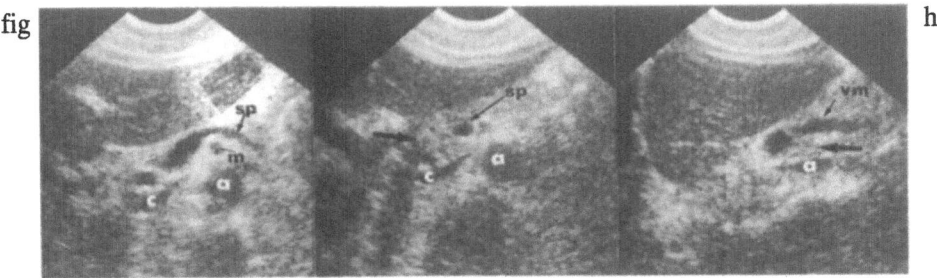 h

Fig. 1.1.f, g Transverse pancreatic section *s* = Uncinate process (↓) is retrovenous (*sp* = splenic vein, *m* = superior mesenteric artery, *c* = vena cava, *a* = aorta), **h** sagittal section: the uncinate process (↓) appears posterior to the mesenteric vein *(m)*

In principle, our mass appears to be a pancreatic carcinoma. But in principle only, since a histologic diagnosis can never be reached on the evidence of ultrasound alone. For the histologic diagnosis ultrasonically guided puncture is necessary. One final morphologic question before we study the diagnostic strategy required by this mass: there is an echogenic strip directly anterior to the tumoral mass (Fig. 1.1a below); to what does that correspond?

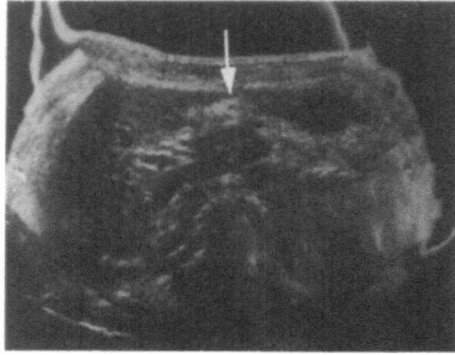

Fig. 1.1a

It's the falciform ligament.

Analysis of the liver tissue is obviously indispensable in the diagnosis of this tumoral process. There is no metastasis: the image of the falciform ligament should not be confused with a pathologic element.

Are any additional procedures necessary?

If we hold with the notion of a metastatic pleural effusion, surgery does not appear justified. If we do not, the right time for a biliary by-pass (preventive intervention, or intervention only after the onset of jaundice) may be discussed. Cytohistologic proof of the malignant nature of the mass should be sought by guided puncture.
If there was no evidence of pleural metastases, the following should be carried out successively:

● Guided puncture to confirm the diagnosis of malignancy. The prognosis of a pancreatic mass of this size is unquestionably fatal. Its resection should perhaps not be considered at all. An inflammatory mass, however, would justify resection.
● A CT scan to precisely evaluate the local extension of the mass; the eventual decision to operate will depend on the results of the scan.
● There is no indication for an arteriography here. The sonogram shows compression of the splenoportal confluence. Contrast enhanced CT will show any collateral channels or even direct involvement of the splenic vein.

1.2. Now that you have thoroughly analysed the pancreatic lesion in the preceding case, study Fig. 1.2 below. Two parallel transverse scans were performed on Mr. Plum, whose condition has changed for the worse. Going from Fig. 1.2a to Fig. 1.2b there is little change in the appearance of the aorta *(a)* and vena cava *(c)*. In Fig. 1.2b the spinal canal is visible (white arrow), whereas it is masked in Fig. 1.2a by a vertebra. The appearance of the spinal canal (↓) shows that the two sections are separated by an interval of two to three centimeters. Was scan 1.2b performed higher or lower than scan 1.2a?

a 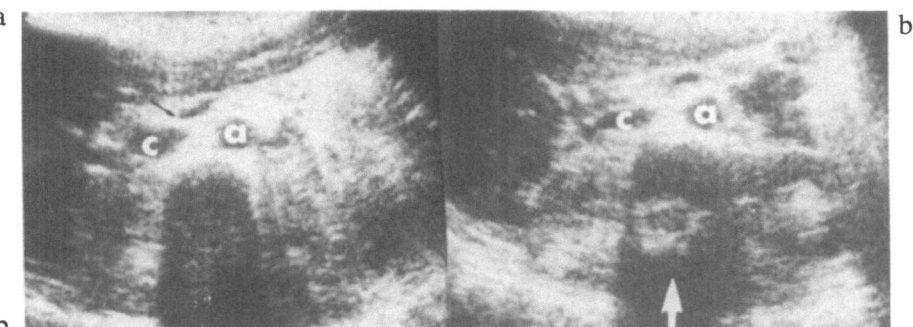 b

Fig. 1.2

Look at the splenoportal confluence in Fig. 1.2a (black arrow). In Fig. 1.2b below, it is not the elongated confluence which has been cut through, but the superior mesenteric vein itself, the cross-section of which is more rounded (‡). So we are at a lower position. Note the uncinate process (↓) curling around the posterolateral wall of the mesenteric vein. Certainly you have spotted a mass (Fig. 1.2b above). This sonolucent prerenal mass has scalloped edges (open arrow, Fig. 1.2b below).

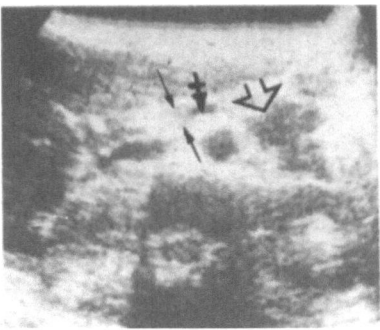

Fig. 1.2b

This is the typical image of? . . .

... of carcinoma of the body and tail of the pancreas.

Wrong! Such images are frequently seen is this area. They are due to the section of a segment of the transverse colon. Examine your patients in an upright position, lengthen the real-time examination, repeat the examination 1/2 to 1 hour later, and take into account only those images which do not change during these expanded examinations. In this way, you'll cure many of your patients of pancreatic tumors which, happily, they never had.

In the rare cases where such images persist, a CT examination will help.

Chapter 2

Six Painful Hepatomegalies

Mrs. Juniper (Fig. 2.1), Mr. Aspen (Fig. 2.2), Mr. Elm (Fig. 2.3), Mr. Sycamore (Fig. 2.4), Mrs. Holly (Fig. 2.5) and Mrs. Ashe (Fig. 2.4) complain of pain in the right upper quadrant. Clinical examination reveals varying degrees of hepatomegaly in all six patients.

2.1. Mrs. Juniper has had dull pains for several weeks. During the clinical examination, the hepatomegaly is clearly evident; there are bulges on the anterior surface of the liver.

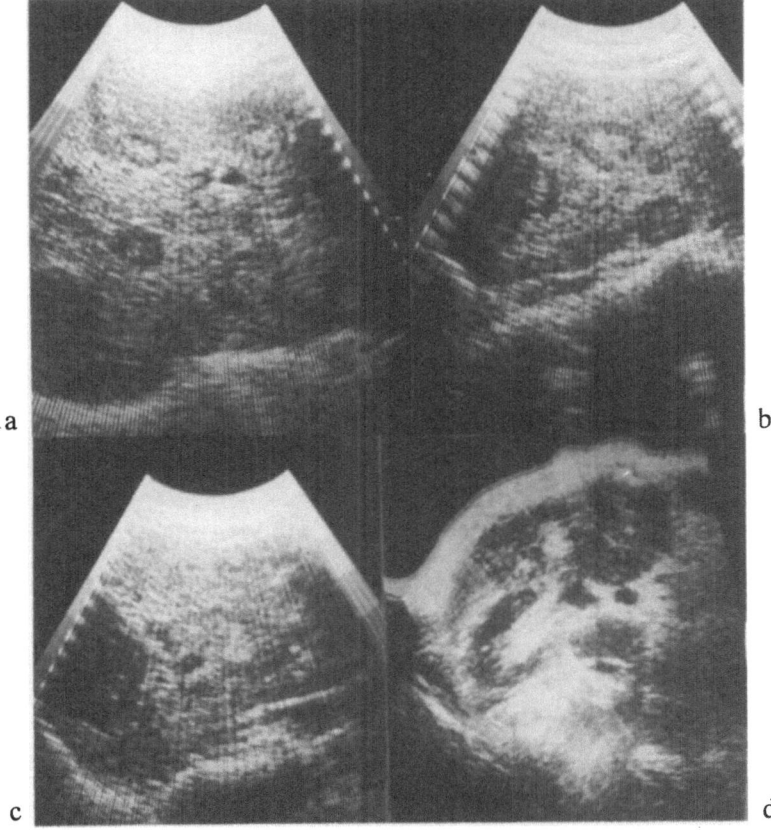

Fig. 2.1. a Recurrent oblique section, **b, c** intercostal sections, **d** transverse section

Transverse section 2.1d explains the nodular character of the liver surface (see preceding page, then below). A tumoral mass (black arrows) is expanding within the caudal part of the left hepatic lobe. It pushes the abdominal wall (white arrows) forward and comes into contact with the great vessels (a = aorta, c = vena cava) behind.

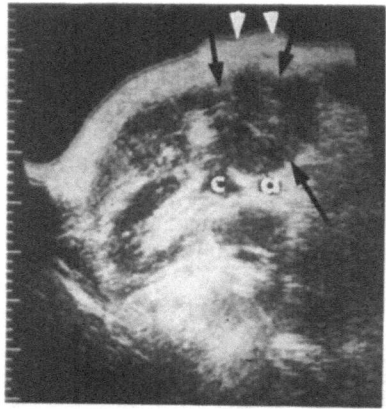

Fig. 2.1d

A reflecting nodule (↓ below) is seen in contact with the external part of this tumoral mass. Does it correspond to a metastasis?

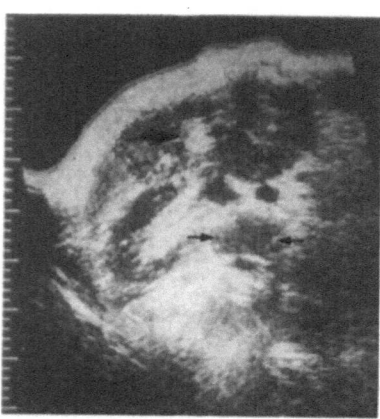

Fig. 2.1d

Most unlikely: it is the...   ... falciform ligament.

From an anatomical point of view, what does the element designated by horizontal arrows in Fig. 2.1d above correspond to?

It's a vertebral body.

12

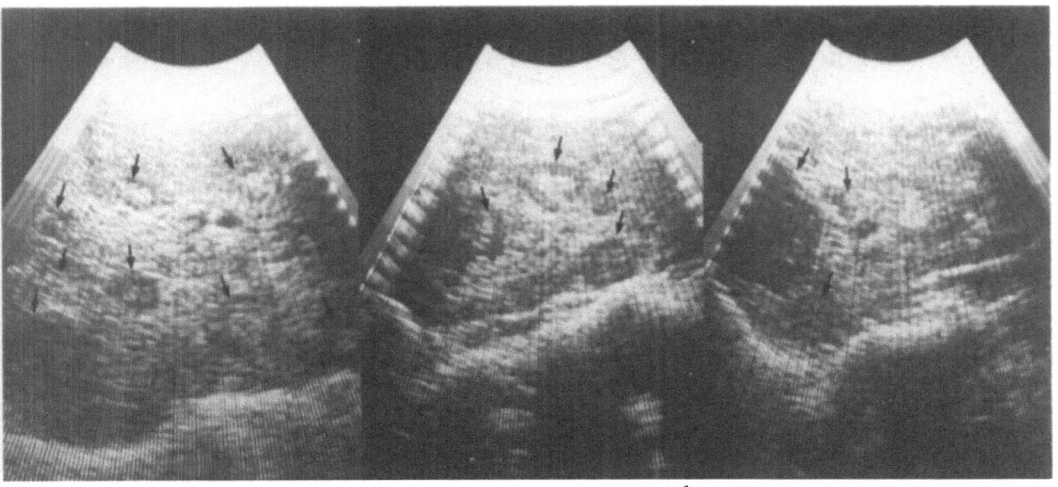

Fig. 2.1   a   b   c

The solid mass discovered in the left hepatic lobe may lead us to consider quite a number of tumoral processes, benign or malignant. But look again at Fig. 2.1a–c on page 11 and above.

We see multiple nodules (↓) which are mostly target-like in appearance. The diagnostic hypotheses can therefore be narrowed down. The only benign process which can be considered is that of multiple hamartomas[1]. In fact, these are typical images of multiple metastases. Hepatomas may be multinodular but usually show fewer regular bull's-eye patterns. If the primary tumor is identified, no other procedure should be considered, with the possible exception of arteriography as a prelude to intra-arterial chemotherapy.
If the primary lesion is not known, if it does not appear on ultrasound sections, and if the diagnosis is important for a therapeutic decision, the best complementary procedure is ultrasonically guided puncture.
In this case the nodules were metastases from a colonic carcinoma; they constituted the first clinical manifestation of the disease.

---

1 Recently acute mycotic abscesses have been described with this pattern (P. Cooperberg, personal communication)

2.2. Mr. Aspen. In this patient a painful anterior hepatic protrusion is found on palpation, which the figure below (Fig. 2.2a–c) will explain.

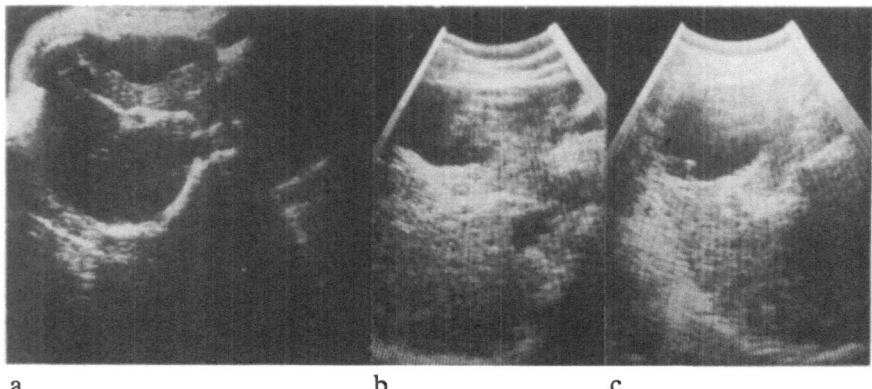

Fig. 2.2. a, b Transverse section, **c** sagittal section

Transverse section 2.2a shows that the bulging corresponds to an intrahepatic collection close to the anterior border of the liver (white arrows below); pressure on this area results in localized pain. This image of collection is also found in sections 2.2b, c (↓). It is well delineated; the liquid pattern is obvious.

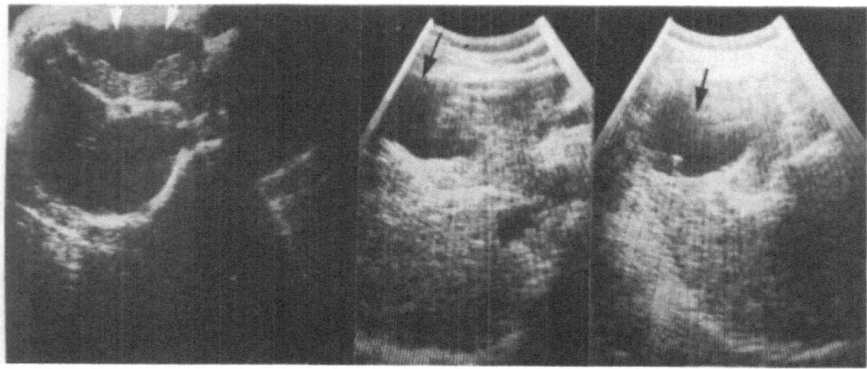

Fig. 2.2

Sagittal section 2.2c shows a small posterior zone of parietal thickening (↓ below).

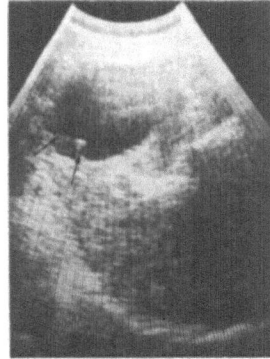

Fig. 2.2c

What will the diagnostic hypotheses be?

● A necrotic metastasis? But the limits of such metastases are usually more irregular, with thick walls (Fig. 2.2d, arrowheads, below).

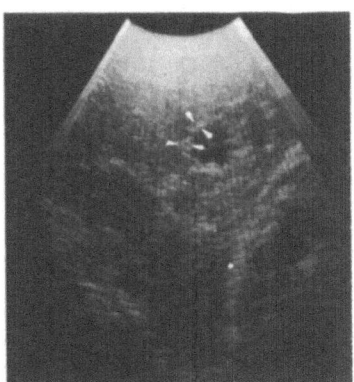

Fig. 2.2d

In fact, necrotic metastases can take on a pseudocystic appearance, especially during the course of chemotherapy.
The clinical data are not in favor of a *cystic tumor* such as a biliary cystadenoma.

● A bacterial abscess? Such a process is possible, but in this case there is no intense fever. In addition, bacterial abscesses often have thick contents, sometimes including microbubbles. Scattered intracavitary echoes with attenuation would mask the distinct posterior reinforcement seen in this case. Unquestionably here, the intracavitary fluid has low attenuation. The small posterosuperior zone of parietal thickening may be part of a localized septum. An infected congenital or biliary cyst is unlikely: the lesion is flattened and there is no proper wall image.

● Now is the time to ask the patient if he hasn't been out birdwatching in the Amazon, since such a collection is consistent with

an complicated echinococcal cyst

or, more likely, an amoebic abscess.

The clinical aspect of these two conditions may be unspecific. Fever may be absent in the case of amoebic abscesses. Once mature, these lesions are often quite sonotransparent, as in this instance. They may actually occur without the patient having a history of exotic travel. Echinococcal cysts are found in many countries of the temperate zone.

So, what's to be done?

It is not recommended to puncture echinococcal cysts. Just in case, a vial of hypertonic saline solution should always be handy when puncturing a cystic lesion.

We shall rely on the biological tests and only puncture a collection which may correspond to an amoebic abscess. If the diagnosis is then confirmed, we can hope the abscess will heal with medical treatment, especially if already emptied and drained under ultrasonic guidance.

In addition, once an echinococcal cyst is ruled out, puncture will confirm the less frequent diagnoses considered above, namely necrotic or cystic tumor and infected cyst.

In Mr. Aspen's case, the collection was due to an amoebic abscess.

2.3. Mr. Elm's clinical history is more or less the same as Mr. Aspen's, except that there is no localized swelling. For many years, Mr. Elm has reared dwarf crocodiles on the banks of the Green Nile for use in ladies's handbags.

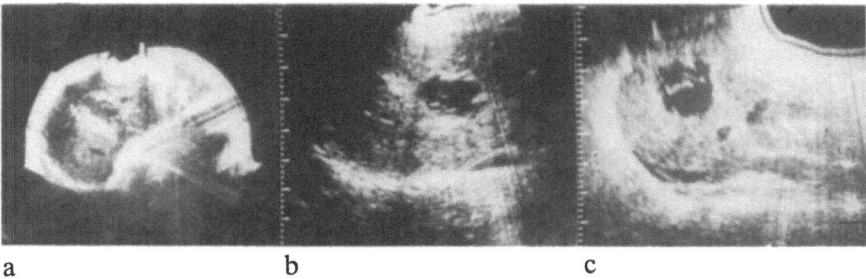

a   b   c

Fig. 2.3. a Transverse section, **b** intercostal section, **c** sagittal section

Sections 2.3a, b (below) show a central hepatic cavity with irregular borders (↓) and small intracavitary foci (white arrow).

a 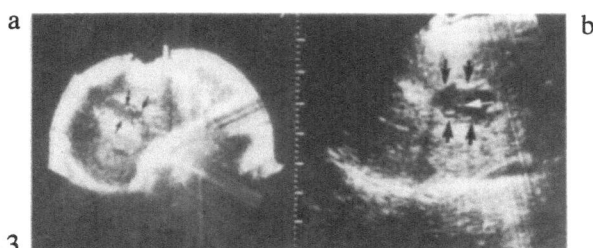 b

Fig. 2.3

Sagittal section 2.3c reveals an intracavitary septum (arrows).

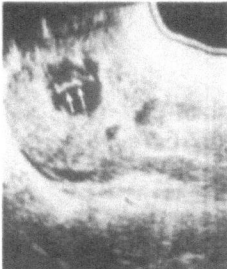

Fig. 2.3c

This image is highly indicative of an aging echinococcal cyst where the membrane is becoming detached. What procedures should be carried out to advance in the diagnosis?
First a CT scan in order to detect parietal calcifications[1]. Since immunological tests will confirm the diagnosis of echinococcal disease, we shall not puncture this cyst.

---

1 Regarding large calcified foci, ultrasound is more sensitive than plain X-rays

What other septated cystic lesions can also be encountered in the liver? (Cover the following list while your think).

- Congenital cysts
- Exceptional multilocular metastases, mainly due to malignant mesenchymomas
- Cystic cholangiocarcinomas
- Biliary cystadenomas
- Cavernous hemangiomas

In fact, such lesions have a multilocular pattern rather than irregular septations as in this case.

2.4. Mr. Sycamore has lived life to the full. In other words, he has secured the benefit of a regular and repetitive exogenous coronary vasodilation, and managed to maintain an elevated blood level of vasodilators for forty years. Unfortunately, he has not only succeeded in dilating his coronary arteries, he seems also to have dilated his liver, which now clears the costal edge. This hepatomegaly appeared rapidly and is painful.

A sagittal section (Fig. 2.4) shows that the liver, while palpable, is not greatly enlarged; discordance between echographic and clinical findings is not rare. This is a ptosed, retracted liver, where attenuation in depth is increased (↓ below). These are typical cirrhotic features.

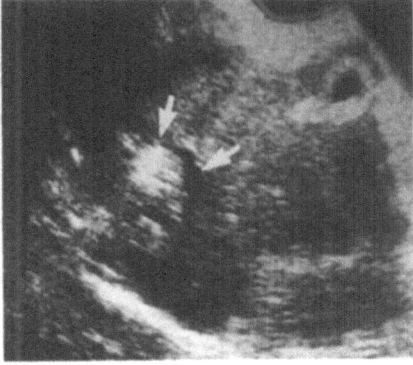

Fig. 2.4. Sagittal section

You have noted a large nodule near the hepatic dome (white arrows, below).

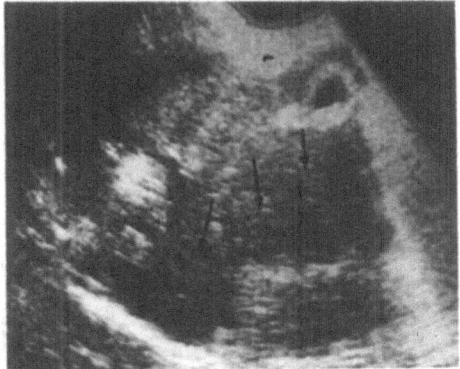

Fig. 2.4

It is an echogenic nodule with irregular borders, more or less displaying a bull's-eye configuration.

19

In such a liver, this tumoral image obviously suggests a hepatoma. But we must not forget the very obviousness of the diagnosis demands histological control, which can be carried out with guided puncture if...? (answer below[1]).

What do you think about the gall bladder? (Fig. 2.4, previous page).

It is abnormal (open arrow below).

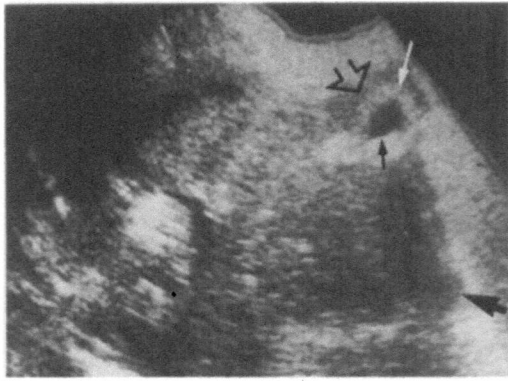

Fig. 2.4

A thin layer of dependent sludge (small black arrow) casts a shadow (black arrow). This indicates the presence of a microlithiasis. There is also a frank thickening of the gall bladder wall (white arrows). Your diagnosis, then, will be that of...?

...acute cholecystitis.

However, palpation under real-time control is painless. From a clinical point of view, there is nothing to suggest acute cholecystitis. Actually, the gall bladder wall may show a thickening of non-inflammatory origin.
Gall bladder wall thickenings may be caused by:

● Acute or subacute cholecystitis
● Chronic cholecystitis
● Acute hepatitis
● Gall bladder carcinoma
● Parietal edema, related to ascites
● Parietal edema due to stasis (resulting from renal or cardiac failure, for instance or to lymphatic obstruction)
● Hypoglobulinemia

---

1 ...if coagulation is not altered and ascites not abundant

Obviously, the appearance of this lithiasitic gall bladder is not that of carcinoma. The absence of pain counts against acute cholecystitis, and we are dealing with a cirrhotic patient. Thus, the possibility of ascites must be checked. Indeed, that is the case here (Fig. 2.4 below). The effusion appears above the hepatic dome (white arrows). It is also visualized between the liver and gall bladder on the one hand and the perirenal fat on the other, i. e. in Morison's pouch (crossed arrows).

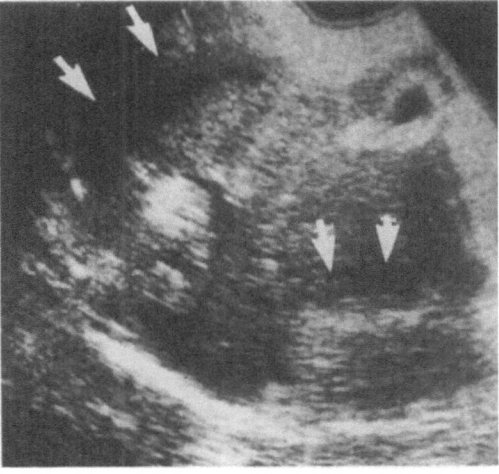

Fig. 2.4

As in this case, detection of thickened gall bladder wall, when there is no previous history of acute inflammation, often leads to the discovery of ascites, which may be of very small extent.

Now we know why this retracted rather than enlarged liver is palpable like a hepatomegaly. It is a floating liver, pushed away from the liver dome by abundant ascites.

2.5. Mrs. Holly has a hepatomegaly. It is painful, spontaneously and on palpation. The hand detects a bulging liver.

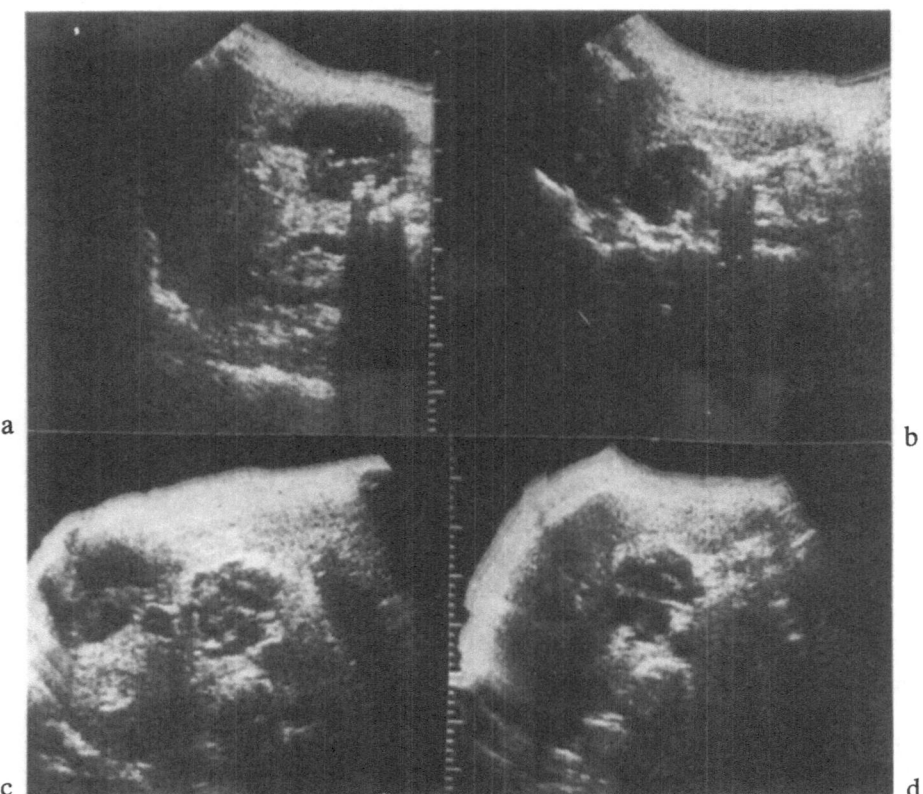

Fig. 2.5. a, b Sagittal sections, c, d transverse sections

The sagittal section in Fig. 2.5a shows a highly complex lesion responsible for the hump detected on palpation (black arrows below).

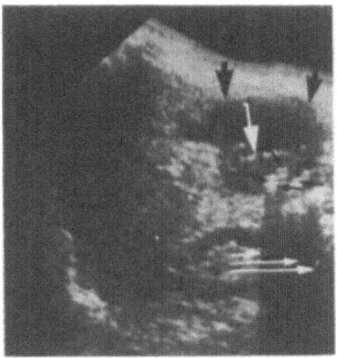

Fig. 2.5a

This lesion is obvously related to the gall bladder, which is highly abnormal. It is enlarged and contains a few dependent stones (small black arrows) which give rise to 'organ pipe' acoustic shadows (thin white arrows). A level of separation within the gall bladder lumen (large white arrows) indicates sludge and stasis. The posterior gall bladder wall in the vicinity of the kidney and the adjacent posterior infundibular wall are abnormally echogenic and thick.

The presence of sludge suggests gall bladder hydrops. Lithiasis and localized parietal thickenings may indicate associated subacute cholecystitis. However, the localized character of the thickening does not tally with that interpretation. Thus, the possibility of carcinoma must be a first consideration.

If we now look at the transverse section (Fig. 2.5c below), we find this abnormal gall bladder (arrows) between the liver and great vessels (a = aorta).

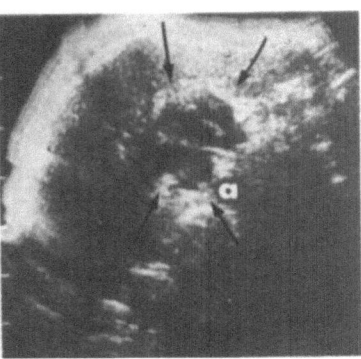

Fig. 2.5c

Moreover, a sagittal section (Fig. 2.5d) shows a partially necrotized mass (curved arrow below) in the adjacent liver tissue. A small independent nodule (↓) is displayed between the two structures.

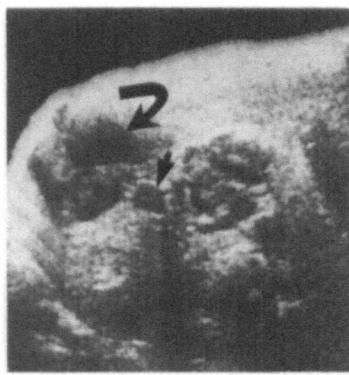

Fig. 2.5d

At this stage in the discussion, our diagnosis must be gall bladder carcinoma with liver deposits. The extent of these lesions puts them beyond surgical therapy. We can, however, confirm the diagnosis of malignancy by guided liver puncture. Computer tomography would also contribute to a better analysis of the tumoral extension. In this elderly patient, however, it is probably not advisable to carry out other procedures.

But is that all there is to say?

Like kremlinologists, we should scrutinize not only that which is seen, but also what is not seen.

It is surprising that a gall bladder tumor of this size, extending to the infundibulum, has not yet invaded the biliary confluence. No section shows a dilation of the intrahepatic bile ducts. We have grounds, then, to consider the liver mass to be indeed a metastasis and not the result of a direct spread.

2.6. Mrs. Ashe is also suffering from a painful hepatomegaly.

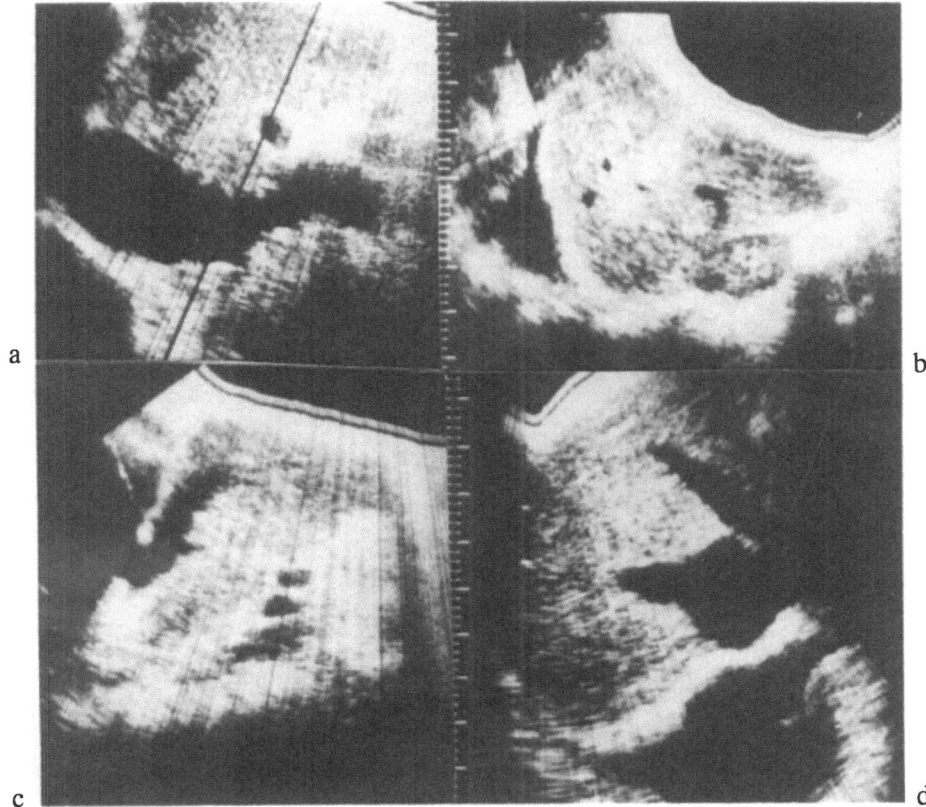

Fig. 2.6. a–c Sagittal section, **d** oblique subcostal section

First, let's look at the sagittal section 2.6a.

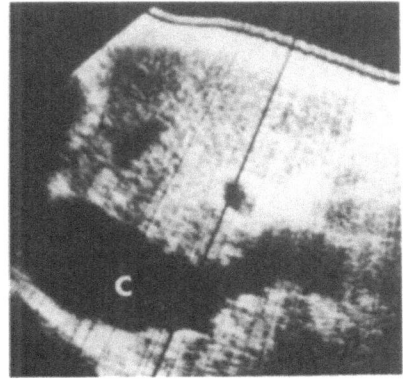

Fig. 2.6a

You should be struck by the abnormal character of the vena cava: the vessel is dilated. A real-time examination showed it to be completely akinetic, without respiratory collapse. Immediately, a diagnosis of venous hypertension by right cardiac insufficiency is suggested. The dilatation is also found at the level of the hepatic veins (Fig. 2.6d, open arrows, below) as seen in an oblique recurrent section. The dilatation of these hepatic veins is also found in sagittal sections (Fig. 2.6a, c). The oblique recurrent section also shows a retrohepatic fluid collection (curved arrow).

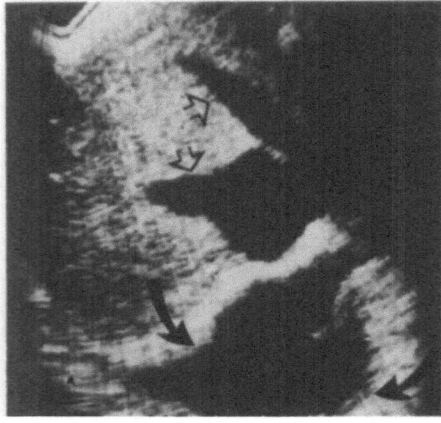
Fig. 2.6d

We have already seen this type of image in Fig. 1.1a, b. It is a right pleural effusion, also clearly visible above the diaphragm in sagittal section 2.6b. In these right cardiac insufficiencies, it is also advisable to check for the possible presence of a small amount of ascites. In addition, we will examine the heart in real time to determine its dilation and kinetics and to check for any pericardial effusion.

Chapter 3

Two Additional Cases of Hepatomegaly

3.1. Mr. Cedar complains of pain in the right upper quadrant. He has lost weight. Palpation reveals an enlarged liver with a smooth surface.

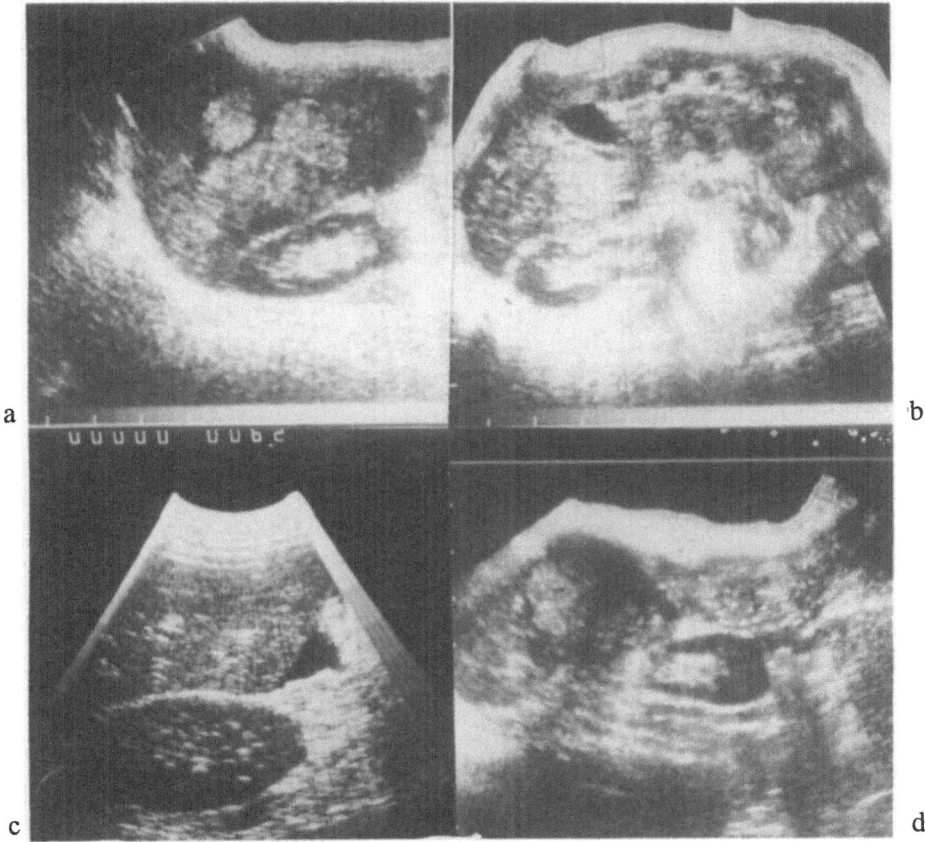

Fig. 3.1. a Sagittal section, **b** transverse section, **c** right intercostal section, **d** coronal section

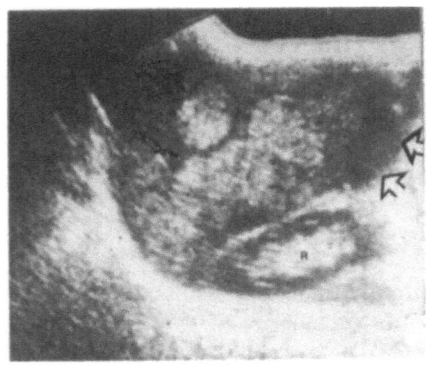

Fig. 3.1a

A sagittal section (Fig. 3.1a above) shows that the liver clearly extends below the inferior pole of the right kidney *(R)*. The echotexture is markedly heterogeneous with echogenic nodules, bull's-eye nodules, and abnormal echogenic fields. The inferior hepatic contour balloons out (edge sign; open arrows) and bulges (hump sign). These are the characteristics of a metastatic liver. The pathologic nature of the left lobe also appears in the coronal section (Fig. 3.1d, p. 27).

The transverse section 3.1b below...

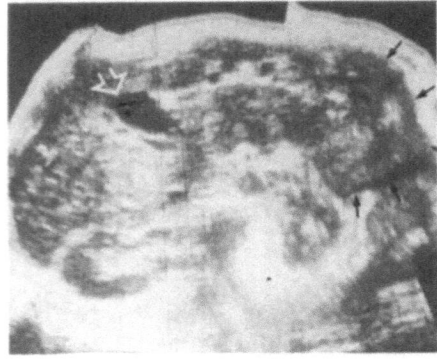

Fig. 3.1b

...confirms the large hepatomegaly, particularly of the left lobe, whose external border (↓) is abnormally rounded. The oval sonolucent field within the right lobe obviously corresponds to the transverse section of the gall bladder (open arrow).

But what else?

There is a small fluid strip behind the gall bladder (Fig. 3.1b p. 28, then large arrow below).

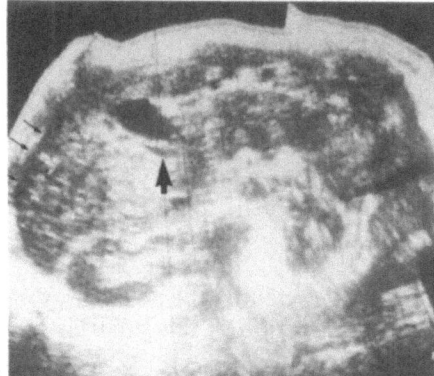

Fig. 3.1b

Ascites is likely to extend between the liver and a gall bladder embedded in a very deep vesicular fossa. Some fluid is seen to the right between the liver and abdominal wall (Fig. 3.1b p. 28, then above, small arrows). This ascites is more clearly seen in the intercostal section (Fig. 3.1c), in contact with the posterior aspect of the liver, between the latter and the undulating limit of intestinal loops (arrow below).

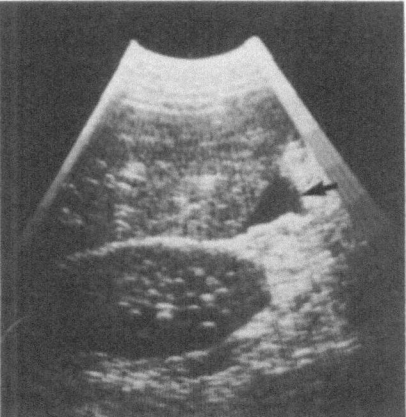

Fig. 3.1c

Can we go away and relax now? Not so fast. Look again at Fig. 3.1b (above, then p. 30).

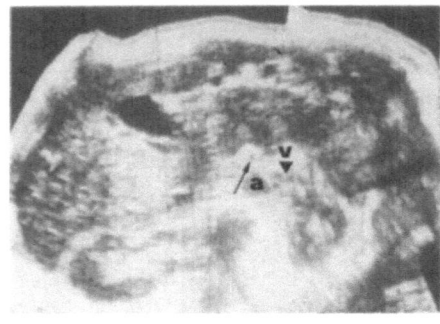

Fig. 3.1b

Here we can identify the aorta *(a)*, the renal vein *(v)*, and anterior to the aorta the transverse section of the superior mesenteric artery (↓). The presence of these vascular elements shows we are at the level of the pancreas. Consequently, the mass (black arrows, Fig. 3.1b below) which is outlined between the superior mesenteric artery and the liver is a pancreatic mass. An inflammatory process could be considered if this mass was the only abnormality, since the ascites could be related to pancreatic necrosis. But, don't forget the hepatic metastases – they confirm the diagnosis of voluminous pancreatic cancer. And if you look again at the liver tissue, you will note a dilatation of intrahepatic bile ducts, distinctly visible in the right lobe, between the perirenal fat and external hepatic contours (small white arrows below).

Before discussing our strategy, one last morphologic question: What does the area of sonolucency marked by an open arrow in Fig. 3.1b (below) correspond to?

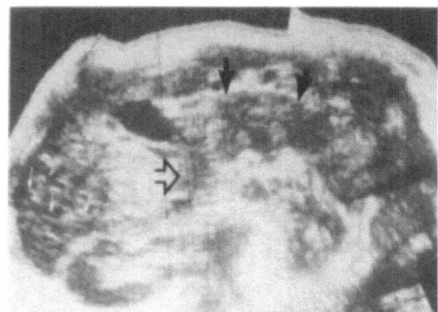

Fig. 3.1b

It is the shadow of a gas bubble in the descending duodenum.

Now let's consider our strategy. If there were no hepatic metastases or ascites, puncture of the pancreatic mass would be called for in order to verify its tumoral nature. Puncture is probably optional in this particular case since, considering the extent of the lesions, it is difficult to envisage an active therapy. Palliative external drainage would be considered after the onset of jaundice. Guided puncture would be justified, however, before intravenous or intra-arterial chemotherapy.

3.2. Mrs. Catalpa complains of swelling. Her abdomen is distended, with the liver participating in this general picture.

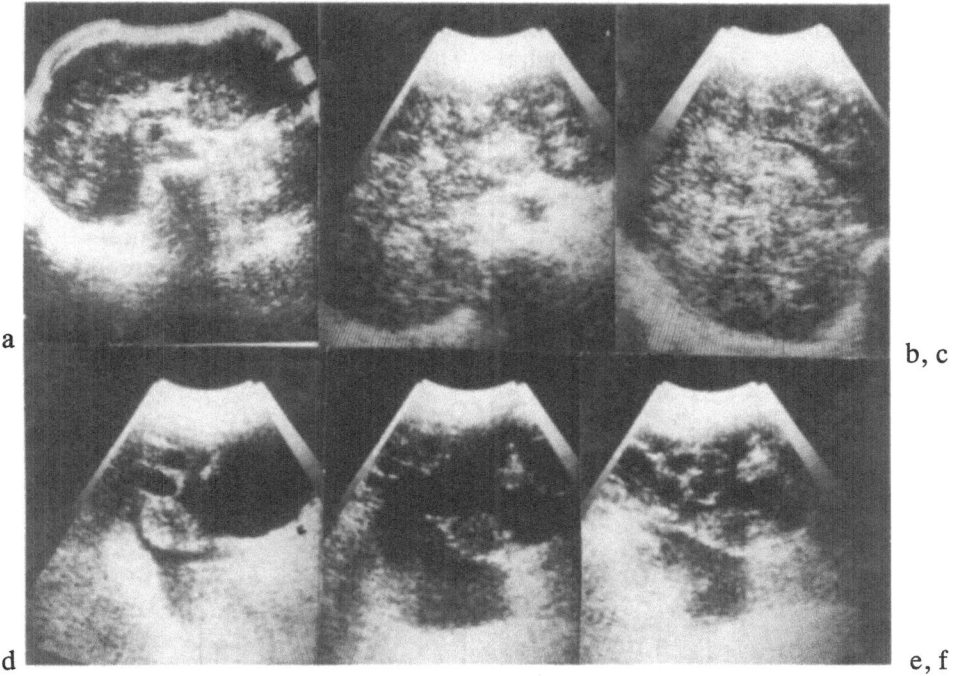

a

b, c

d

e, f

Fig. 3.2. a, b Transverse sections, **c** recurrent oblique section, **d–f** pelvic transverse section

Let's look at the hepatic transverse section (Fig. 3.2a above, then below).

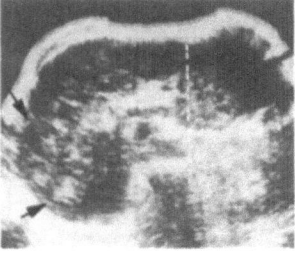

Fig. 3.2a

Is the liver enlarged?

Yes; the left lobe is clearly swollen (tangent sign[1]).

The echotexture is multinodular ($\downarrow$); it is another example of those metastases whose diverse morphological varieties have already been illustrated in several previous cases. We have already broached the differential diagnosis of these disseminated nodular abnormalities. Theoretically, to the problem of multifocal hepatomas and rare benign tumors we should add that of chronic active hepatitis. Alveolar echinococcosis could also be considered, but we shall not dwell on this parasitosis, since it is highly localized geographically in Central Europe and Alaska. The existence of a few bull's-eye images allows us to rule out these two hypotheses.

The multinodular echotexture of the liver is also displayed in the oblique recurrent section 3.2c (below), which also shows a few sonolucent nodules as well as a deformity of the medial hepatic vein (arrow).

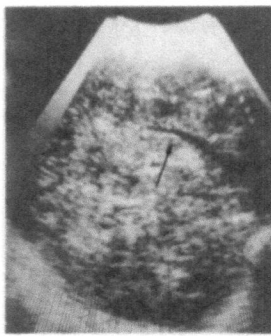 Fig. 3.2c

We now have all the elements necessary to list the different signs of hepatic metastases:

Contour changes
– Hump sign
– Edge sign

Echotextural abnormalities: sonolucent nodules, bull's-eye nodules, echogenic nodules, echogenic fields

What should we look at now?

The kidneys: they are normal. The pancreas: there is no abnormality here either. So we go as far as the pelvis, and study it by parallel transverse sections (Fig. 3.2d–f p. 31, then p. 33).

---

1 The thickness of the left lobe is over 5 cm along the tangent to the left aspect of the spine

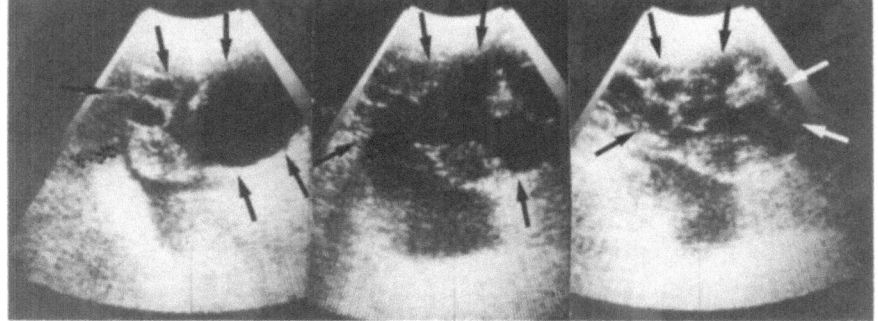

Fig. 3.2

A multinodular fluid collection is observed here (↓). It is tempting to conclude that there is a multinodular ovarian tumor. At this stage in our examination, then, we can consider the diagnosis of ovarian cancer with hepatic metastases, without ascites in the greater sac, and without ureteral compression.

Actually we have moved too fast. Moreover, we have forgotten that it is impossible, after a first macroscopic diagnosis, to formulate a precise diagnosis without cytologic and histologic control. Let us look again at Fig. 3.2e below.

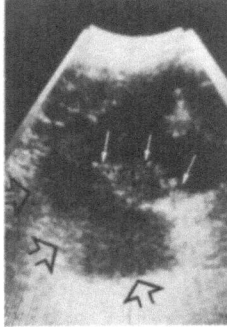

Fig. 3.2e

Doesn't the structure marked by the white arrows remind you of something? It is the classic image of the uterus, prolonged by the broad ligaments, as it used to appear on pelvic X-rays carried out after pneumoperitoneum. The fluid posterior to the uterus (open arrows) is in Douglas' pouch. Obviously, the uterus cannot inhabit an ovarian tumor. What we are seeing, then, is not an ovarian tumor – at least, not a large ovarian tumor occupying the entire pelvis. The multilocular structure is that of a septated ascites indicating pelvic metastases of unidentified origin. It is not due to uterine cancer. With the fluid contrast of the ascites, a uterine cancer extending beyond the organ's limits would be identifiable.

What is to be done now?

The next logical step is a coelioscopy with biopsy, and a barium enema (or sigmoidoscopy).

The final diagnosis was cancer of the sigmoid colon with peritoneal and liver metastases.

Chapter 4

A Geological Chapter

Mr. Spruce, Mrs. Palm, and Mrs. Magnolia complain of pain in the right upper quadrant.

4.1. Mr. Spruce is not only feeling bad; he also has a moderate fever. A right parasagittal scan is performed. The liver is normal in the area of the section, but obviously . . .

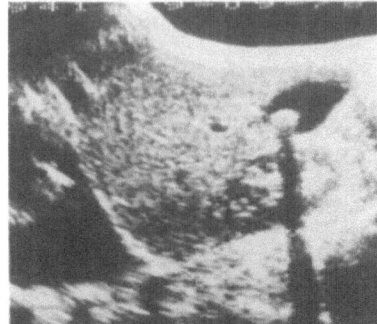

Fig. 4.1

. . . there is an infundibular cholelithiasis (↓, below) with a handsome acoustic shadow posterior to the stone (open arrow).

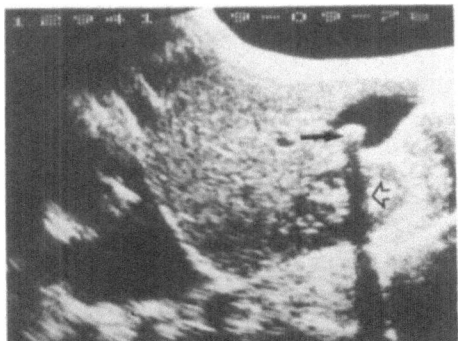

Fig. 4.1

Is the fever related to an inflammation of the gall bladder?

In principle, no: there is neither dilatation, nor stasis, nor...?

...nor thickening of the gall bladder wall.

Now you should ask the sonologist a few questions: Did the transducer's application trigger pain? Was palpation of the gall bladder painful under real-time control? For Mr. Spruce, the answer in each case is no.

Why the fever?

You have no doubt noticed...

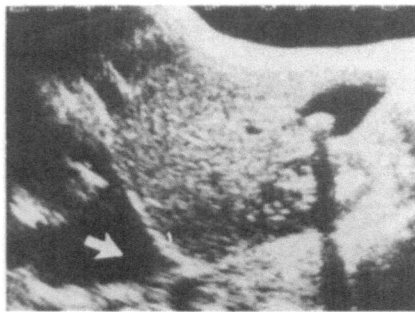

Fig. 4.1

...a pleural effusion (↓ above), marked by the presence of a supradiaphragmatic sonolucency, posteriorly limited by the thoracic wall, which normally is not visible. Absence of dilatation of the hepatic veins, of which certain segments are necessarily cut in this paramedial section, as well as evaluation of the vena cava, show it is not an effusion of cardiac origin. We can hold the lithiasis responsible for the pain, but this patient also exhibits a pleuropathy.

1 a) Morison's pouch. b) Perihepatic recesses. c) Juxtavesicular region. d) Perisplenic region. e) Lesser sac. f) Paracolic gutters. g) Douglas' pouch

4.2. Mrs. Palm is also experiencing pain on the right side.

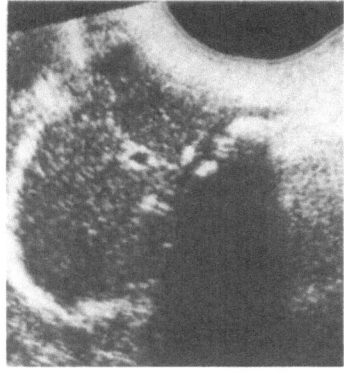 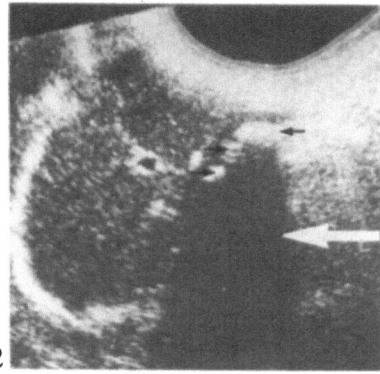

Fig. 4.2   Fig. 4.2

This sagittal section eloquently shows a lithiasis, this time with multiple stones (↓ above) casting a broad acoustic shadow (white arrow). Thus in this geological chapter you have unearthed some new stones.

The thickness of the gall bladder wall is normal. The gall bladder is not particularly sensitive on palpation. Thus there is neither objective nor subjective sign to indicate cholecystitis.

Let's go on the next case.

Not so fast you say, and you're right: there is still something important to be seen...

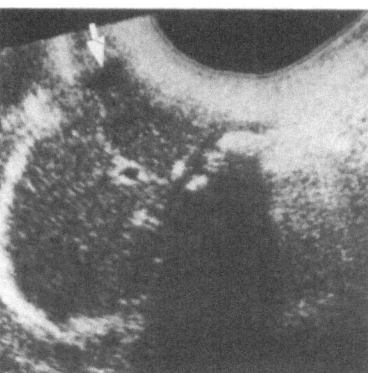

Fig. 4.2

We find a small fluid effusion in the most anterior part of the subdiaphragmatic area (↓ above).

We will confirm the presence of this ascites by examining other sensitive areas which you should enumerate before checking below[1].

Consequently, we are confronted with a diagnostic problem much greater than the simple lithiasis discovered earlier. Actually, it was carcinoma of the ascending colon, unrecognized at that point, with peritoneal spread.

4.3. Mrs. Magnolia also has pain on the right side. She has a moderate fever.

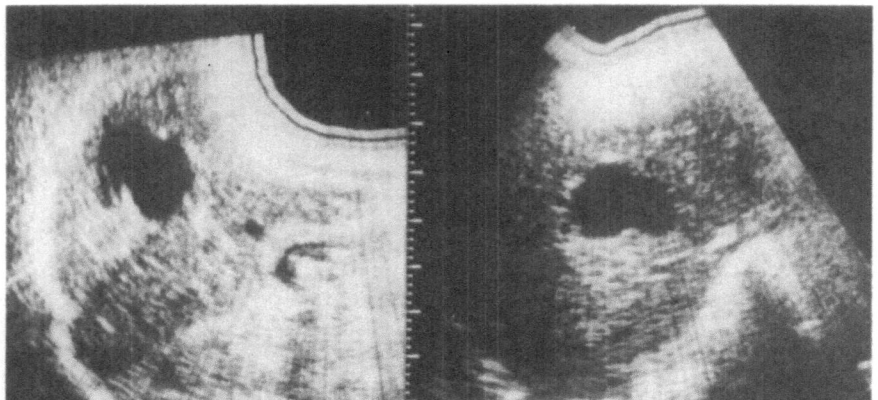

a   b

Fig. 4.3. a sagittal section of right upper quadrant, **b** transverse section

Certainly you have seen the large fluid-filled cavity in the left hepatic lobe (Fig. 4.3a, b; open arrows, below).

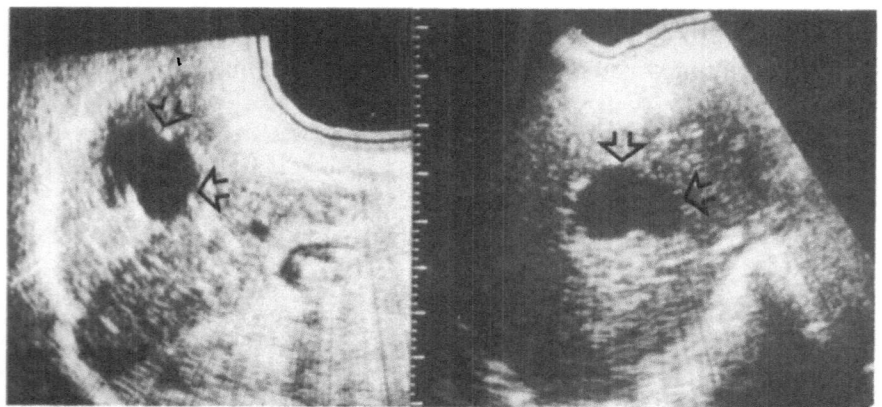

a   b

Fig. 4.3

Is this cavity responsible for the clinical syndrome? Possibly! But also . . .

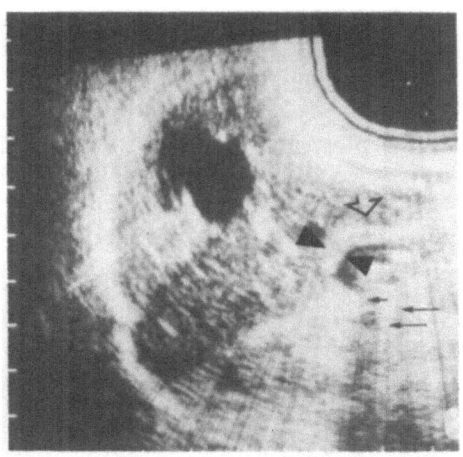

Fig. 4.3a

...the gall bladder is abnormal (open arrow, above). It is small, and filled with stones; organ-pipe shadows are projected posterior to them (↓). The gall bladder wall is thick (arrowheads) and has a sonolucent rim; finally, the transducer triggers pain.

We must then consider acute inflammation (pain, thick wall) supervening on a chronic cholecystitis (small, retracted, lithiasic gall bladder). What does the intrahepatic cavity correspond to? It may be a necrotized metastasis. It may also be a cystic tumor, a cavernous hemangioma, an abscess, a parasitic cyst, a banal serous cyst, or one of those biliary cysts often shown by sonography and CT.

Contrast-enhanded CT may be carried out. A peripheral blush will be in favor of a necrotized or cystic tumor, a prolonged blush in favor of a cavernous hemanioma. CT may also detect, in an echinococcal cyst, peripheral calcified foci too small to appear on conventional X-rays. After having ruled out echinococcal disease and angioma, we will puncture, either during surgery, or, if a cholecystectomy is not immediately considered, under ultrasound guidance. In liver angiomas fine needle puncture does not necessarily cause hemorrhage but has poor cytologic results.

In this case the fluid was clear. The final diagnosis was plain benign cyst.

4.4. Mrs. Willow is suffering – you guessed it – from pain in the right upper quadrant and discreet hyperthermia. Distant colleagues, still unfamiliar with the virtues of sonography, had her undergo an intravenous cholangiography without results.

While analysing these ultrasonic documents including four longitudinal and one transverse section of the gall bladder, keep in mind that longitudinal scan 4.4d was performed with the patient upright.

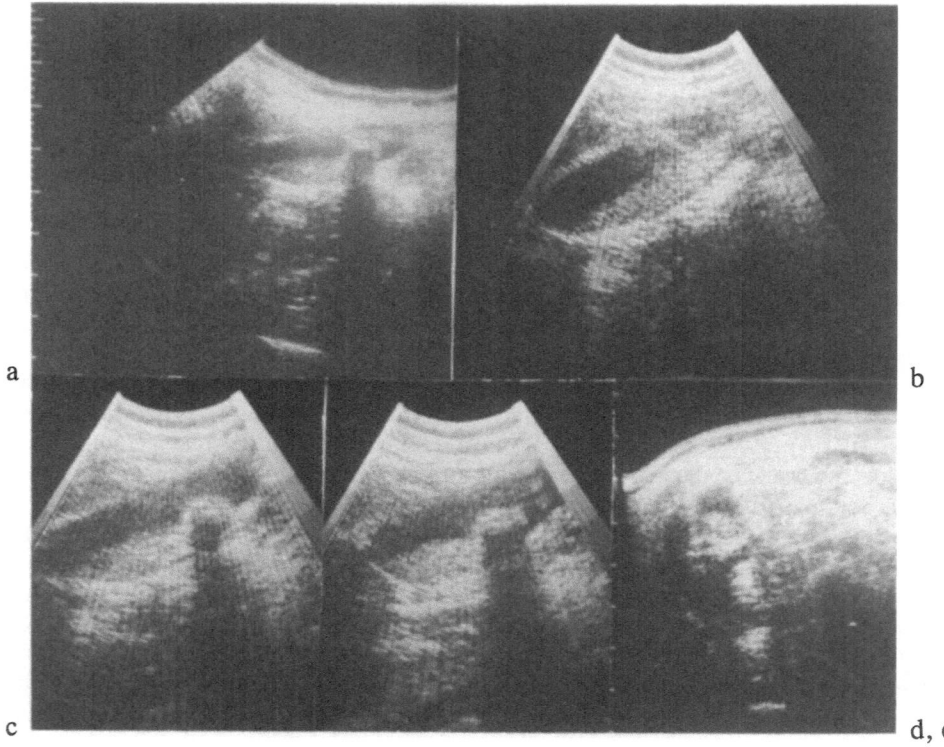

Fig. 4.4. a–c Longitudinal sections, **d** longitudinal section (in upright position), **e** transverse section

This gall bladder is large and contains a large stone (Fig. 4.4a, c below). The reflection on its anterior aspect causes a shadow which masks its central and posterior part, and also the adjacent gall bladder wall.

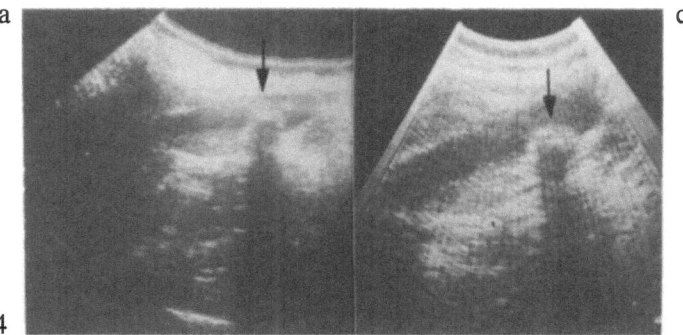

Fig. 4.4

Well, what else?

There is also a dependent echogenic strip, visible in each cut (4.4a–e ↓ below).

What does it correspond to? To biliary sand?

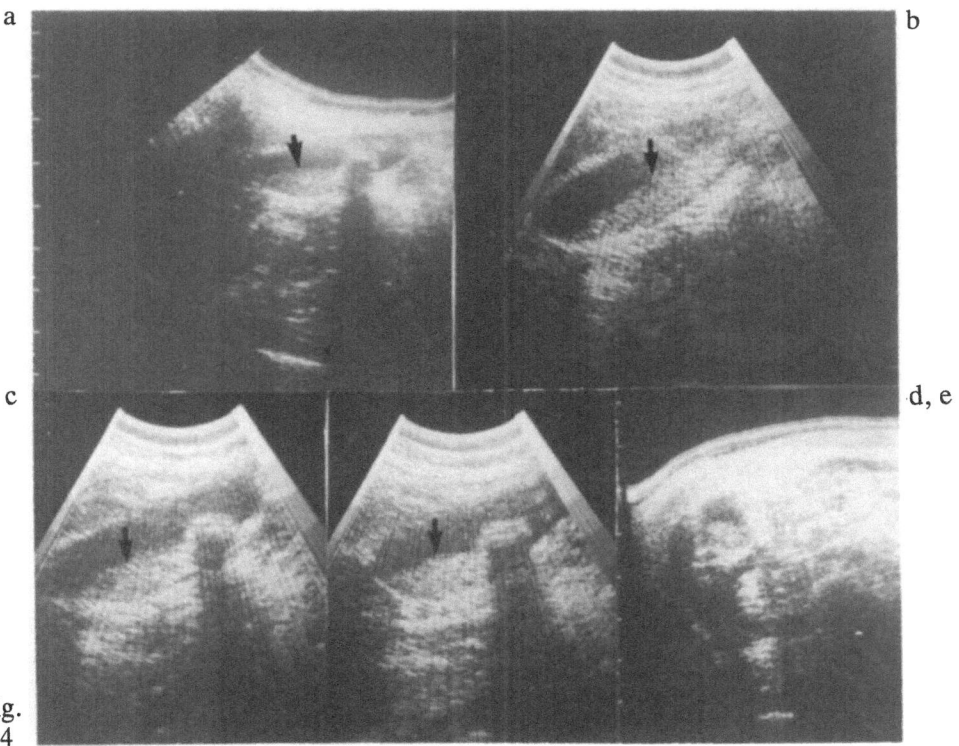

Fig. 4.4

That is not likely. If the strip was caused by such a thickness of microlithiasic sediment there would be an acoustic shadow. Above all, the standing position (Fig. 4.4d) should cause this echogenic sediment to shift to the bottom of the gall bladder. A new fluid-solid level, perpendicular to the previous one, would appear. In this case the orientation of the sediment and level of separation does not change when the patient is placed in standing position. Thus the sediment is sludge, rich in cholesterol crystals.

We can deduce that the gall bladder, which is enlarged, does not empty.

We are dealing, then, with gall bladder hydrops with stones.

The cystic blockage is not visible in these sections.

Something else should draw your attention in the positional scan (Fig. 4.4d).

In standing position, the large gall-stone which should have shifted to the gall bladder bottom, remains in the same position, indicating an impaction. This is a sign of parietal inflammation. Is this process also apparent in the gall bladder wall? Yes, the wall is thick. This is particularly evident in the transverse section (Fig. 4.4e below ↓).

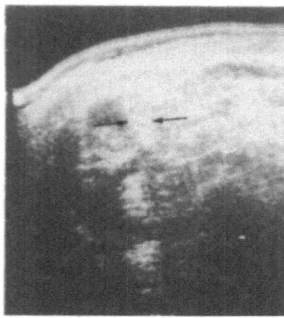

Fig. 4.4e

It is so evident that we can answer: "Gall bladder hydrops with stones and objective signs of acute cholecystitis," confirmed by triggered pain.

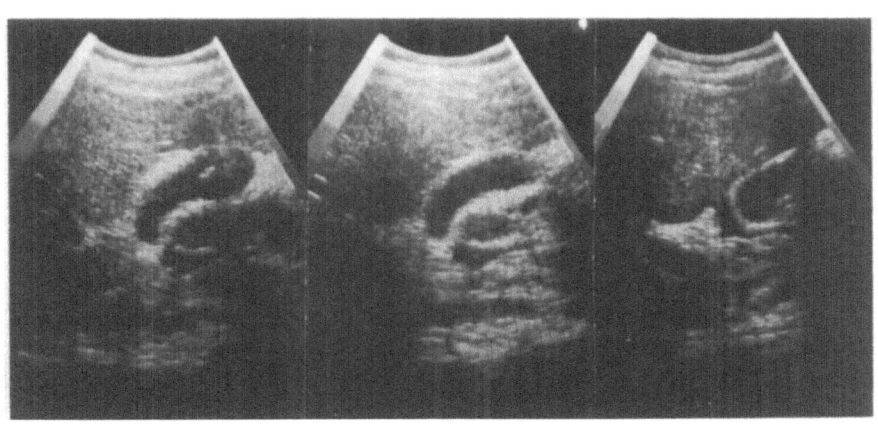

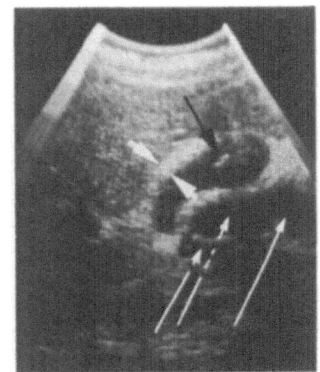

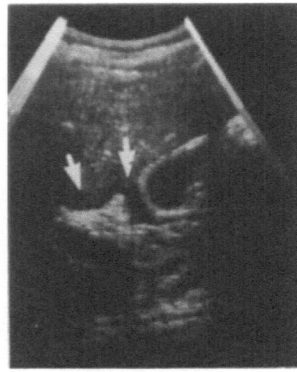

Fig. 4.5b

Fluid is also demonstrated around these collections (white arrows). What we are
seeing then, are dilated fluid-filled intestinal loops, caused by a paralytic ileus and
floating in an intraperitoneal effusion. The presence of a paralytic ileus is not
surprising in this picture of acute cholecystitis; but proof of distinct peritoneal
involvement indicates it is time to sharpen up those Swiss knives.

4.6. Mrs. Hickory is suffering from the same syndrome as Mrs. Dogwood.

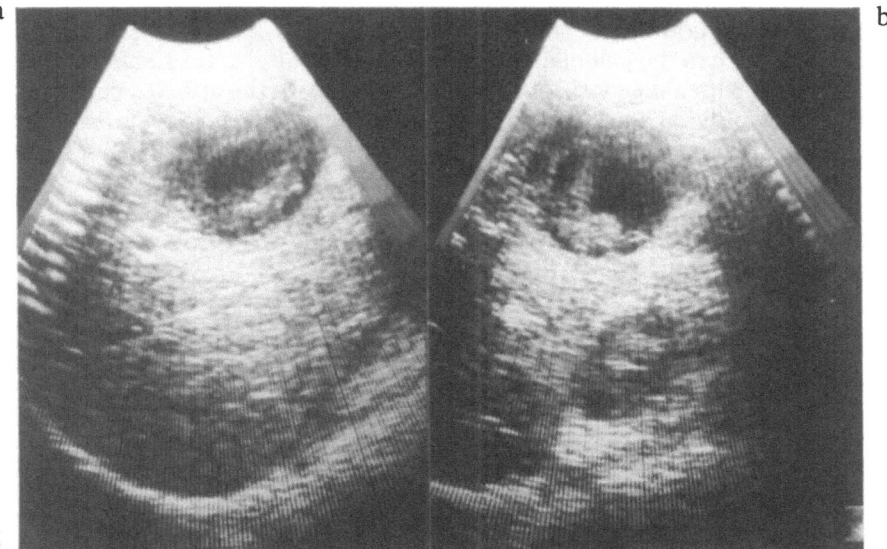

Fig. 4.6

Palpation under real-time control causes elective pain. What do the two parallel parasagittal sections (4.6a, b) show?
They show a considerable thickening of the gall bladder wall (arrowheads, Fig. 4.6a, b, below) as well as a small dependent deposit (↓) which seems to be sludge rather than sand.

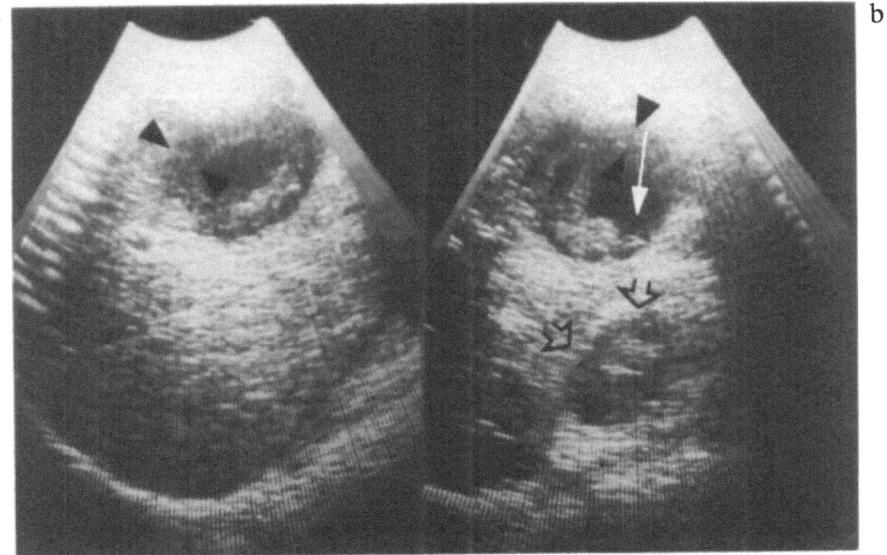

Fig. 4.6

What does the bull's-eye nodule posterior to the gall bladder (open arrows, Fig. 4.6b) correspond to? We might consider a hepatic lesion; actually, it's simply a marginal section of the right kidney. This is readily recognized during the real-time examination.

Let's go back to the gall bladder. In this clinical pattern, thickening of the wall is consistent with a diagnosis of acute cholecystitis. In the absence of pain, such an image of parietal thickening might suggest gall bladder carcinoma. In acute cholecystities, a thickening this great may be consistent with gall bladder empyema, with risk of a juxtavesicular abscess. Echogenic foci within the thickened wall represent gas bubbles.

So you were quite correct in noticing the beginning of a purulent intraparietal and juxtaparietal collection (↓ Fig. 4.6a, b below).

a

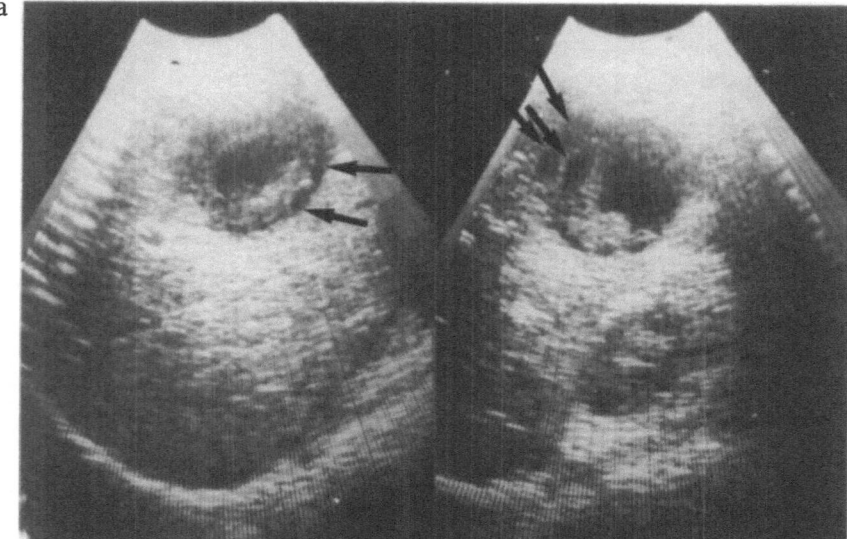

b

Fig. 4.6

This abscess is still restricted: in analysing the renal image (Fig. 4.6b) you have noticed the absence of fluid in Morison's pouch. However, as in the preceding case, intervention is urgent. Now, please list the causes of gall bladder wall thickening (answer in footnote[1]).

---

1 Acute cholecystitis, chronic cholecystitis, acute hepatitis, carcinoma, ascitic edema, edema due to stasis of cardiac and renal origin, hypoglobulinemia, other infiltrating processes

4.7. Mr. Balsam is a nice young man, but a bit yellowish.

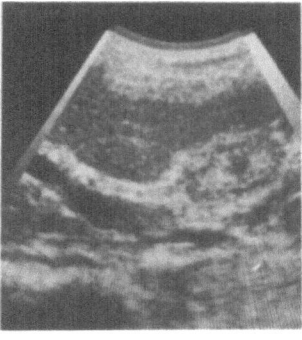 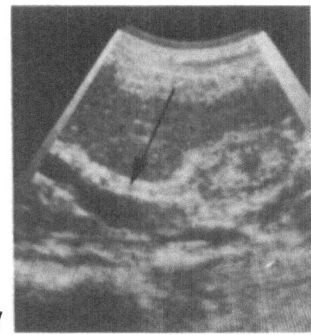

Fig. 4.7

Fig. 4.7. Intercostal section

Clinical and biological results are unclear: Is it hepatitis? An obstructing syndrome? An intercostal section of the right upper quadrant (Fig. 4.7 above) shows a normal bile duct. It appears anterior to the portal vein as a fine ductal structure (arrow).

What do you think of the gall bladder?

Its wall is thickened, and it is also physiologically abnormal: only the central part of the lumen remains sonotransparent. In fact the gall bladder is completely filled with sludge (open arrow, below).
Look at Fig. 4.7b below. You will find a layer of sludge ($\downarrow$) comparable to that found on p. 40. You can easily reconstruct the mechanism by which the other image (Fig. 4.7) was formed.

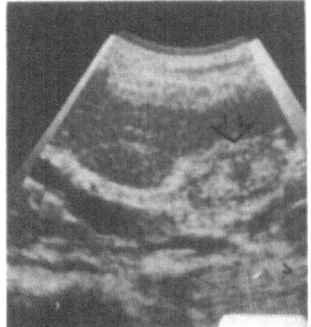 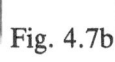 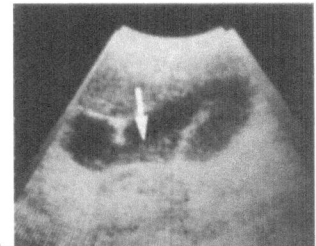

Fig. 4.7   Fig. 4.7b

The occurence of sludge does not necessarily indicate an obstruction of the cystic canal. Physiological stasis due to parenteral alimentation or pregnancy may suffice.

Ultrasound examination of this patient shows no sign of obstruction. He has hepatitis, which can also induce wall thickening[1]. A fat-free diet has modified the gall bladder appearance; its image returned to normal with normal alimentation.

---

1 Here are the different causes of gall bladder wall thickening, already mentioned: bacterial and viral cholecystitis, carcinoma, edema (ascitis, cardiac or renal failure), hypoglobulinemia

4.8. Now that you have become eminent geologists, you will wonder perhaps what kind of problem could be posed by the images taken from Mr. Hemlock (Fig. 4.8a) and Mr. Mapel (Fig. 4.8b), who are both suffering from pain in the right upper quadrant.

Well?

a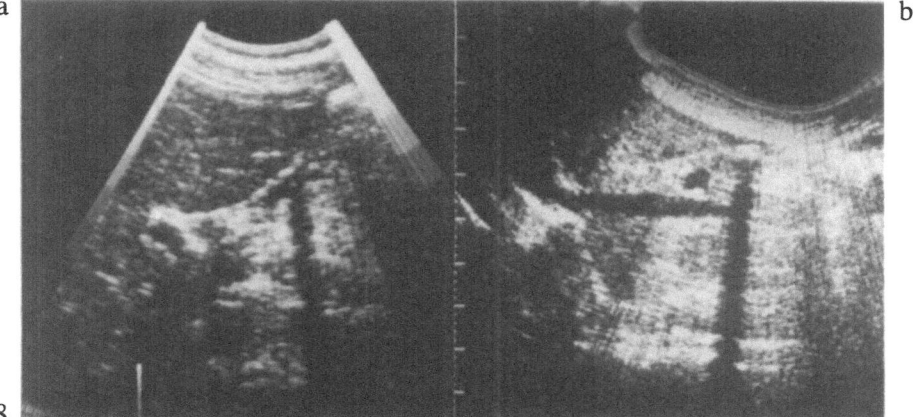b

Fig. 4.8

Well, the image from Mr. Hemlock (Fig. 4.8a), contrary to that from Mr. Mapel (Fig. 4.8b), is not one of lithiasis with acoustic shadow (arrow, below).

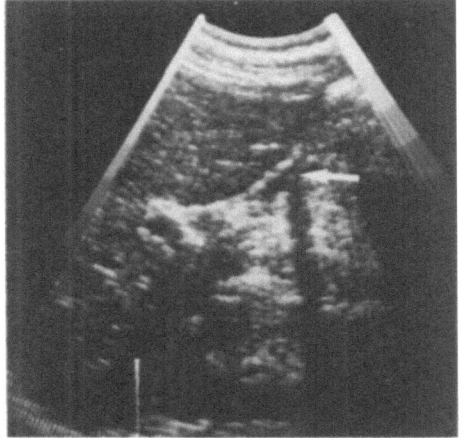

Fig. 4.8a

It's a common pitfall, related to an air bubble trapped in part of the digestive tract – here, the duodenal bulbus. Contrary to what has been published by eminent authorities, shadows caused by gas can be as intense and as clearly delineated as those of authentic gall-stones. In order not to make this mistake:

a) Verify the absence of the normal gall bladder image in a fasting patient. As a last resort the gall bladder should be sought by intercostal approach and recurrent oblique scans below the medial hepatic vein and gall bladder fossa.

b) If the gall bladder is not seen, possible variations or the disappearance of the acoustic shadow with positional changes or with successive follow-up examinations should be checked for. A gall-stone shadow is constant while that of a bubble changes.

Another pitfall is the acoustic shadow from the cystic duct, caused by diffraction of the ultrasound beam. You should be generally careful of shadows arising from the border of rounded or curved structures – and such is the gall bladder wall. They should also be sought in a perpendicular section before you find stones which are not there.

Chapter 5

In Which it is Shown that the Ways of the Lord are Unfathomable

For a change of pace, we shall pick up the pieces of Messrs. Tamarack, Boxelder, Sourwood, and Buckthorn.

5.1. Mr. Tamarack had to leave his girlfriend's boudoir in a hurry, owing to an unexpected visitor. Rushing headlong into what should have been a broom closet, he found himself falling from the second floor. He has several fractured ribs on the right side and is in pain.

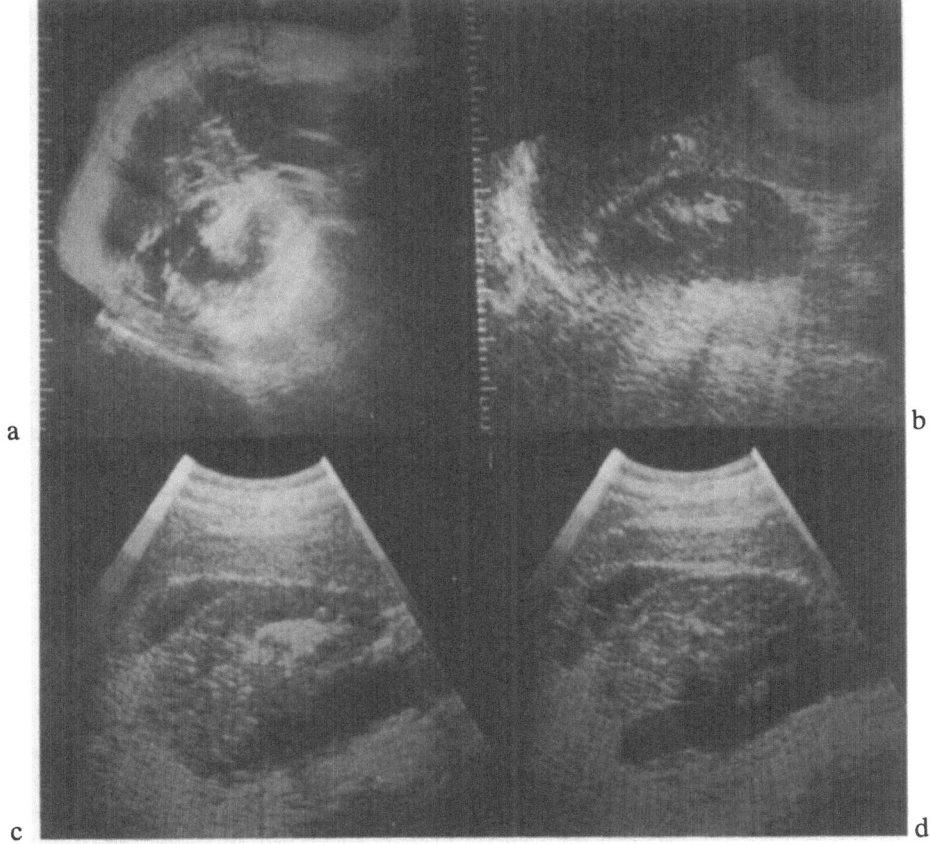

Fig. 5.1. a Transverse section, **b** sagittal section, **c, d** right intercostal sections

A transverse section (Fig. 5.1a) shows us a liver normal in appearance. The kidney *(k)* looks still fit for use, but... what?

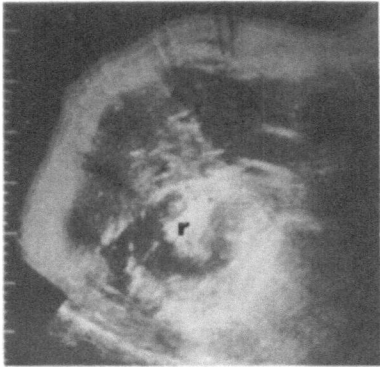

Fig. 5.1a

...But there's a sonolucent band between the lateral border of the kidney and the liver, indicating the presence of fluid (arrows below).

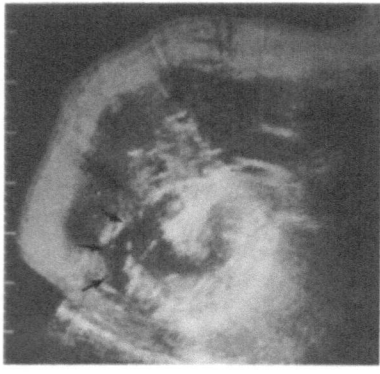

Fig. 5.1a

The location of this fluid may be:
- Hepatic (subcapsular)
- Perirenal
- Pararenal
- Renal (subcapsular)
- Intraperitoneal, in Morison's pouch

Figure 5.1a shows that the fluid is not in Morison's pouch. Effusions in Morison's pouch are found in a more anterior position. The hematoma is therefore either in the perirenal or in the pararenal space. Presence of a thin fatty strip between the kidney and the collection favors a hematoma in the anterior pararenal space.

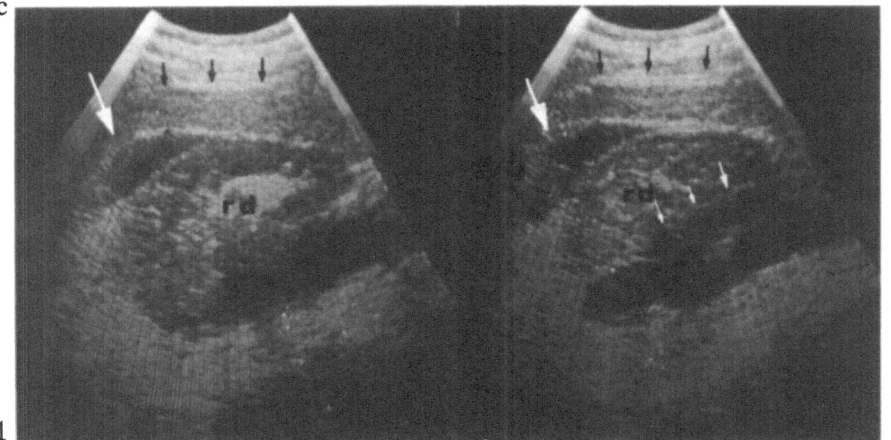

Fig. 5.1

Two parallel intercostal sections (Fig. 5.1c, d, above) also clearly show a subcapsular hematoma (white arrow). It lifts the capsule of the right kidney *(rd)* and overlying perirenal fat, which is limited by Gerota's fascia (small black arrows).

There is also a small strip of intraparenchymatous hematoma (small white arrows, Fig. 5.1d, above). If there was still any uncertainty between hepatic and renal hematoma, it would help to observe the movement of the hematoma in real time. The respiratory mobility of the liver is much greater than that of the kidney. The diagnosis between perirenal hematoma and hemoperitoneum is based on the study of image changes during the respiratory cycle and especially during positional changes. A hemoperitoneum is modified under these conditions whereas a subcapsular hematoma retains the same appearance.

What are the locations of the hematomas indicated by black and crossed black arrows (Fig. 5.1c, d below)?

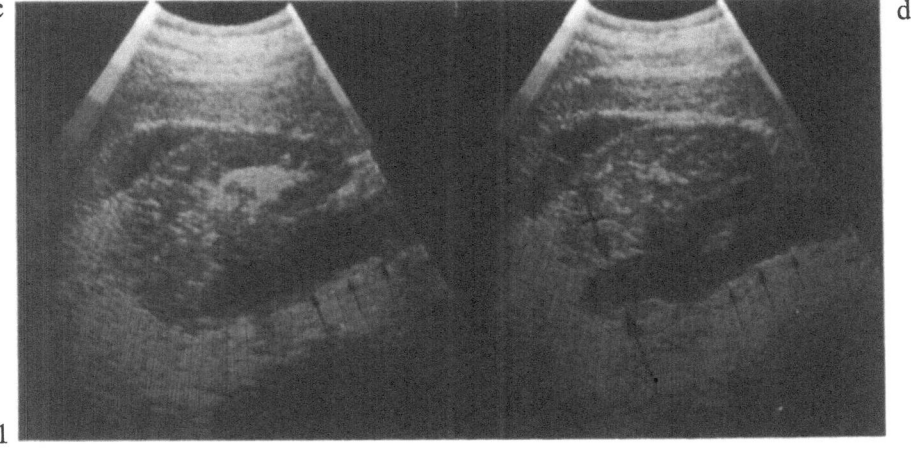

Fig. 5.1

The hematoma indicated by crossed black arrows is in direct contact with the capsule of the kidney; it is therefore perirenal. That marked by the uncrossed black arrows is separated from the kidney by a fatty strip which extends caudally. It must then be considered as being in the posterior pararenal compartment: the location of a collection in the peri- or pararenal compartment can be deduced from its relationship to Gerota's fascia or the renal capsule, and also from its caudal extension, since the pararenal compartment extends further caudally than the perirenal compartment.

We still have to study the sagittal section (Fig. 5.1b, p. 51). How many collections does it show? Two? One? The answer is one: a caudal subcapsular hematoma. The sonolucent strip within the renal upper pole is a refraction artifact.

One last question: Where should we look for a possible hemoperitoneum? (answer below[1]).

Of course, a complete examination of the liver will allow us to rule out the hypothesis of an associated hepatic hematoma at a distance from the kidney. Finally, we shall have Mr. Tamarack undergo intravenous urography to verify the renal function: it is impossible to confirm the integrity of the renal artery on the strength of a sonographic evaluation alone (unless a Doppler study is made). If the urography shows neither frank calyceal tear (not probable in the absence of parenchymatous ultrasonic abnormality), nor change in the kidney function, an arteriography should not be performed. Arteriography should be reserved for cases of renal fracture, massive and evolutive hematomas, clear recurring hematurias, and non-functioning kidneys. CT is of course instrumental in the diagnosis of parenchymal tears, hematomas, and arterial lesions. It can then advantageously replace intravenous urography.

In order to test the experience you have acquired, we suggest you take a look at Fig. 5.1e (below) before going on to the next case.

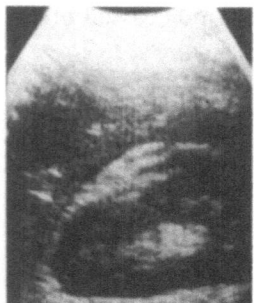 Fig. 5.1e

---

1 In Morison's pouch, as mentioned above, and also in all juxtahepatic recesses, around the spleen, in the lesser sac, in the paracolic gutters, and in Douglas' sac

It is a sagittal section taken in another patient following blunt trauma of the right upper quadrant.
Four distinct hematic collections are present (*1, 2, 3, 4*, Fig. 5.1e below).

Where are these four collections situated?

1 In Morison's pouch
2 Within the anterior pararenal compartment
3 Within the perirenal compartment
4 The last collection is subcapsular
g Gerota's fascia

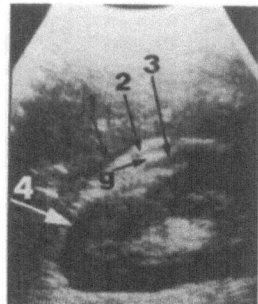

Fig. 5.1e

5.2. Mr. Boxelder has just recognized Mr. Tamarack at the corner of the street following his recent voyage through space.

Since, for more than a year, he has owed the latter some $ 2345 (excluding interest), Mr. Boxelder abruptly changes direction and in attempting to reach a nearby patch of fog, makes contact with the front of an oncoming bus. With a few fractured ribs, he finds himself in a bit of pain.

a 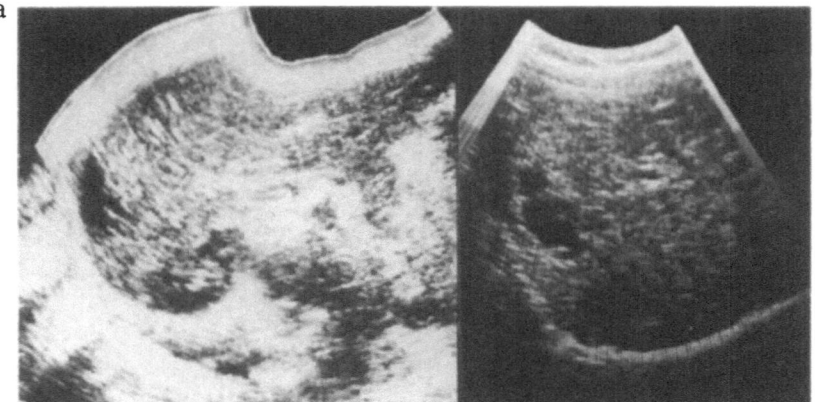 b

Fig. 5.2

On his admission, a transverse section (Fig. 5.2a) and a recurrent oblique section (Fig. 5.2b) show? ...

... a fluid collection which is near the lateral wall of the liver, but clearly intraparenchymal in the recurrent section (arrows, Fig. 5.2a, b below).

This is an intraparenchymal hepatic hematoma. The kidney, retroperitoneal compartment, and peritoneal recesses are checked and no further traumatic lesion or associated blood effusion is discovered.

A lesion of this type calls for arteriography only if there is anemia or if follow-up examinations show an aggravation such as lesional spread, or developing subcapsular hematoma. In such a case, arteriography is more useful than CT.

a 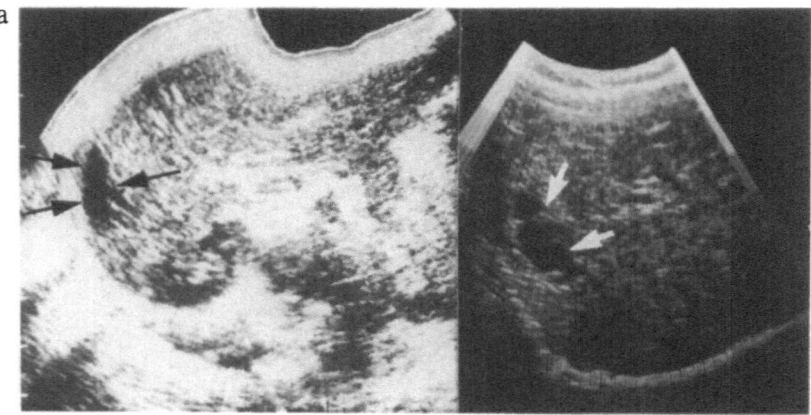 b

Fig. 5.2

56

5.3. Mr. Sourwood is a policeofficer. When he observes Mr. Boxelder hurrying off into the fog, he is convinced he is in the presence of a not too law-abiding citizen: off he goes in hot pursuit. At that very moment the bus driver with whom Mr. Boxelder has entered into conflict hits the brakes in such a way that Mr. Sourwood hurtles into the back of the bus, leaving him with three broken left ribs, not to mention the pain.

On his admission, in the bed next to Mr. Sourwood, intercostal splenic scans (Fig. 5.3a, b) are performed.

a 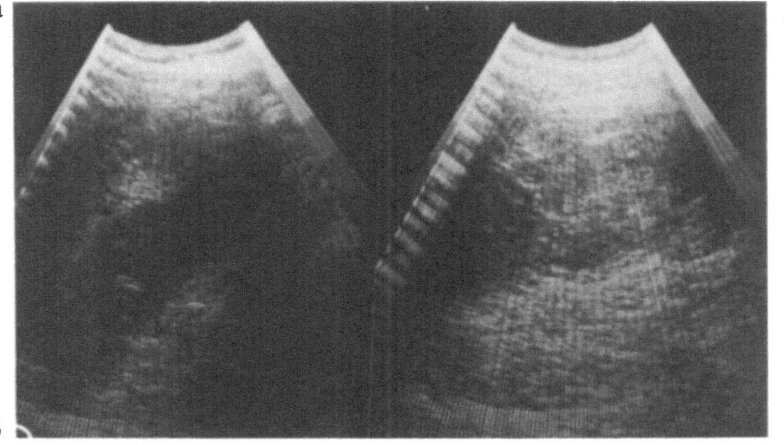 b

Fig. 5.3

They show distinct changes in the splenic parenchyma. You have noted in Fig. 5.3a a triangular, central reflecting zone (arrow, below).

The periphery of the organ, however, is sonolucent.

This image immediately suggests . . . ?

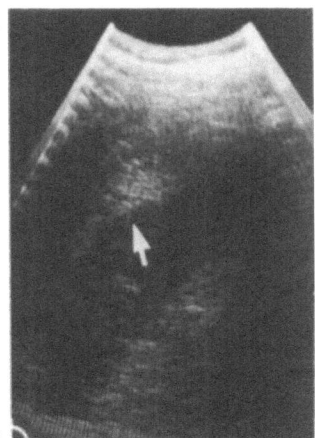

Fig. 5.3a

. . . yes, a large subcapsular hematoma.

The other section (Fig. 5.3b) confirms the heterogeneous nature of the splenic tissue (arrows, below).

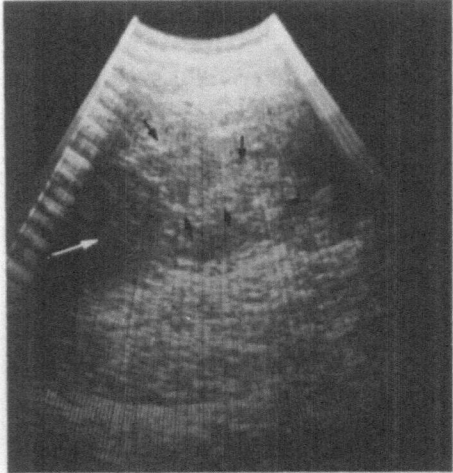

Fig. 5.3b

This is one of those cases of traumatic pathology of the spleen one doesn't discuss too long: we sharpen the scalpels and prime the blood pump. In more discreet parenchymal heterogeneities, without an image of subcapsular hematoma, a more conservative policy is possible.

One may certainly one day come across a previously undetected heterogeneous spleen corresponding to a non-traumatic, pre-existent process. However, the association of trauma, pain, and splenic heterogeneities leaves little room for hesitation, even if the peritoneal washing is negative. Contrast CT can show blood pools within the spleen and images of rupture. In questionable cases, arteriography, while of limited value in small lesions, can be useful. In general, sonography is much more sensitive. Ultrasonic examination of the traumatic spleen naturally includes complementary analysis of the liver, pancreas, kidney, and all peritoneal recesses. These post-traumatic examinations are only easy and reliable in real time, provided a small sector scanner with good image quality is available. Small sector scanners always allow intercostal access, even if the patient is unable to turn. With intercostal approach the study of hepatic, splenic, and renal parenchyma is precise and complete even when there is a paralytic ileus.

5.4. Mr. Buckthorn did not have enough weekends, to practise both gliding and motorcycle riding concurrently, so he satisfied both aspirations at once by executing a glide from his Japanese saddle. He is hospitalized with pain in his right side.

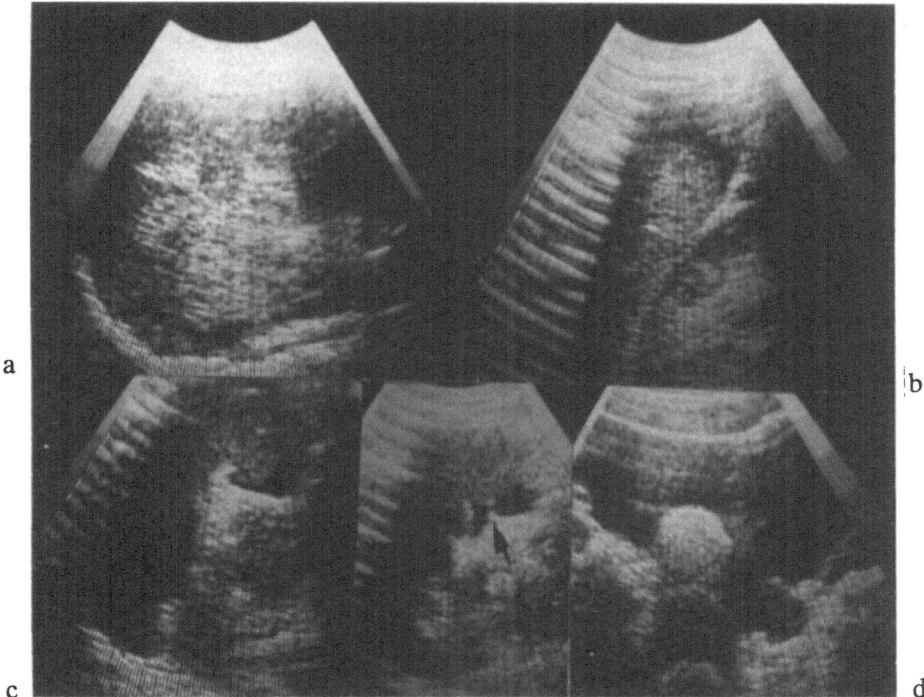

Fig. 5.4.a Right intercostal section, **b–d** left intercostal sections, **e** suprapubic section

The intercostal section of the liver (Fig. 5.4a) shows an abnormal echogenic field indicating a hepatic contusion (arrows, below).

What is the condition of the spleen?

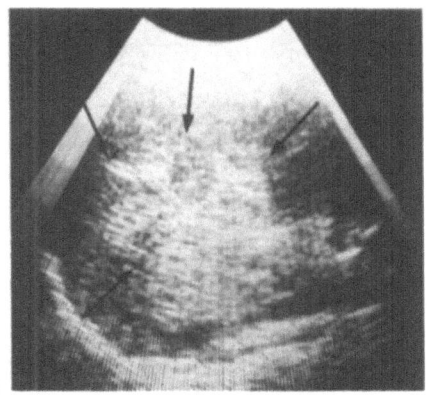

Fig. 5.4a

59

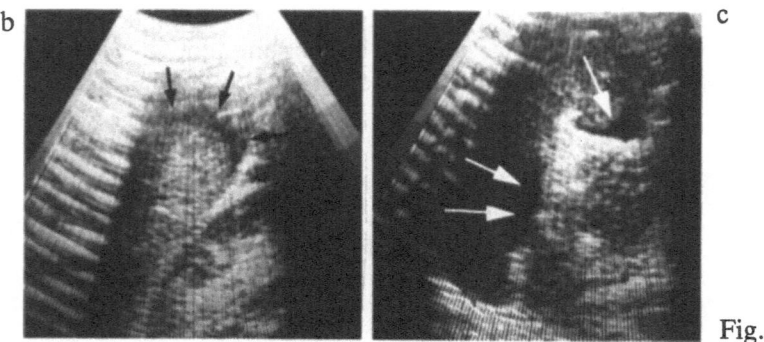

Fig. 5.4

A perisplenic fluid strip is in evidence (arrows, Fig. 5.4b, above).

Does it correspond to a subcapsular hematoma or a hemoperitoneum?

The intercostal splenic section (Fig. 5.4c) above is not decisive.
The answer is found in Figs. 5.4d, e.

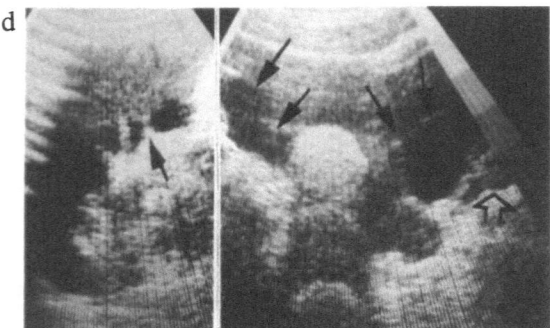

Fig. 5.4

The fluid strip surrounding the splenic hilum (arrows, Fig. 5.4c, above) may be subcapsular. However, in the parallel section (Fig. 5.4d, above) hilar vascular elements are surrounded by fluid (↓). This indicates that the fluid must be intraperitoneal, and not subcapsular. We term this pattern the "flooded hilus" sign.

The suprapelvic sagittal section (Fig. 5.4e, above) also shows intraperitoneal fluid (↓), this time above the bladder (open arrow) and around intestinal loops, confirming the hemoperitoneum.

The combination of hepatic contusion and hemoperitoneum calls for hepatic arteriography. In this case it did not demonstrate hemorrhage. Follow-up examinations showed normalization of the hepatic abnormality and disappearance of the hemoperitoneum.

Chapter 6

A Few Strange, Strange Cases

6.1. Mr. Yucca has lost weight. He also complains of other symptoms, but telling you everything now would make it too easy. Note, however, that his xyphoid process is exceptionally short.

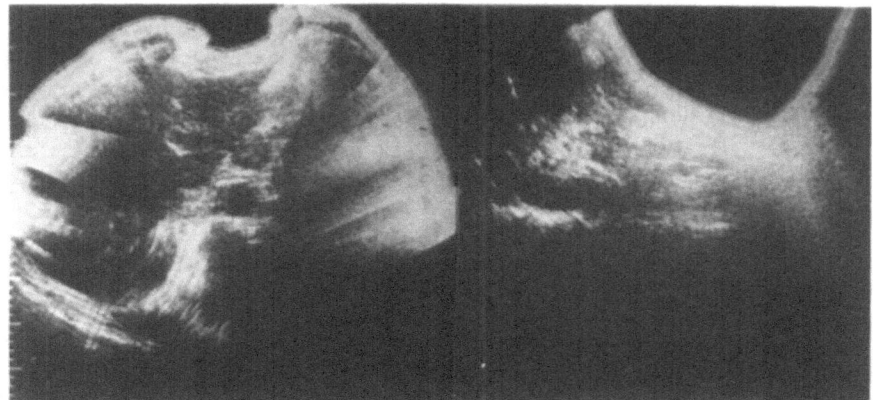

a   b

Fig. 6.1. a Transverse section, **b** sagittal section

A transverse scan was performed in the highest part of the epigastrum.

What does it show?

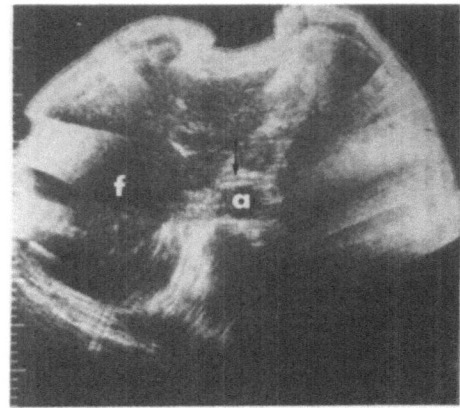
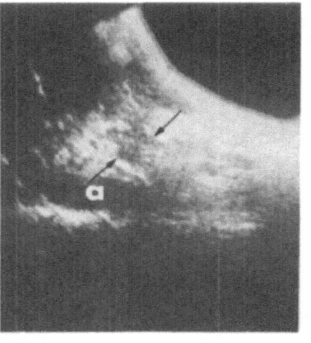

Fig. 6.1

It shows a rounded, preaortic structure (white arrows, above; a = aorta). First, we could consider hypertrophy of the caudate lobe; however, examination in real time has already shown a cleavage plane in relation to the liver. This cleavage plane is clearly visible in this section (black arrow). The mass is also found in the transaortic sagittal section (Fig. 6.1b, arrows, above).

Is it a pancreatic mass?...

...No. Why not?

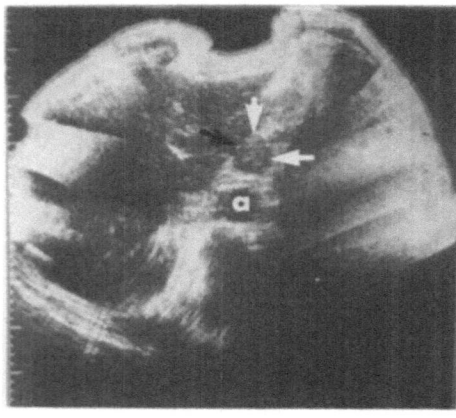

Fig. 6.1a

Careful examination of the transverse section (Fig. 6.1a) shows...
...a fine linear structure curling around the anterior and lateral wall of the aorta (arrow, Fig. 6.1a above).

This linear structure does not correspond to a vessel but to the crus of the diaphragm. Thus, we are at a higher level than the pancreas. In fact, we had already indicated this since the section was carried out high in the epigastrum and Mr. Yucca's xiphoid process is exceptionally short.

In sagittal section 6.1b (below), the pancreatic isthmus (black arrow) is displayed anterior to the mesenteric vein (white arrow). It is caudal to the mass.

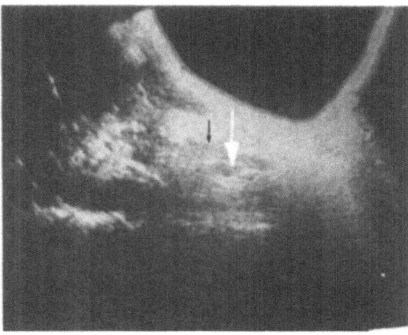

Fig. 6.1b

By the way, you have probably noticed, on this sagittal section, the thin strip of the upper part of the crus of the diaphragm between the mass and the aorta. Where would you find its caudal part? (Answer below[1].) Let's get back to the mass.

We haven't told you the most important clinical fact: dysphagia. In fact, cancer of the lower esophagus was this patient's diagnosis and he was referred for a pretherapeutic ultrasonic evaluation. The liver is free of metastases. This mass poses a problem. Is it an adenopathy or the tumoral mass itself? Is there any way of locating the esophagus? Yes. The patient can be given an effervescent drink to serve as an ultrasound contrast medium. Unfortunately, this usually effective method was unsuccessful in this case.

So finally we had to rely on the conventional esophagogram. X-rays showed a tumor arising from the abdominal esophagus, indicating that the ultrasonic image is that of a primary tumor and not an adenopathy. Like other segments of the digestive tract, the cardiac and fundic regions can be shown in appropriate ultrasonic sections. They are best seen in juxta-aortic sagittal sections. The fundic region has the same appearance as other parts of the empty stomach: a bull's-eye configuration with a thin sonolucent wall. Digestive tumors may appear as unspecific masses or with a thick-walled bull's-eye pattern.

---

1 Posterior to the vena cava regarding the right crus, lateral to the aorta regarding the left one

6.2. Mrs. Walnut is only 35. She has lost a lot of weight. Apart from an elevated sedimentation rate, there is neither functional trouble nor biological abnormality to direct the diagnosis. As soon as the real time head is placed on the abdomen, beginning as always with sagittal and parasagittal sections, a diagnosis can be formulated. What diagnosis?

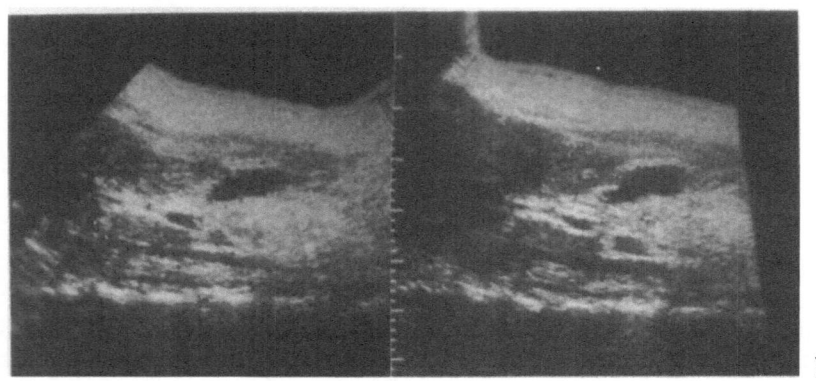

a   b

Fig. 6.2. a, b. Right parasagittal sections

Let's start with an anatomical study.

Two close parallel right parasagittal sections (Fig. 6.2a, b, below) show the gall bladder (open arrow), portal vein *(P)*, bile duct (arrow), and vena cava *(C)*.

a   b

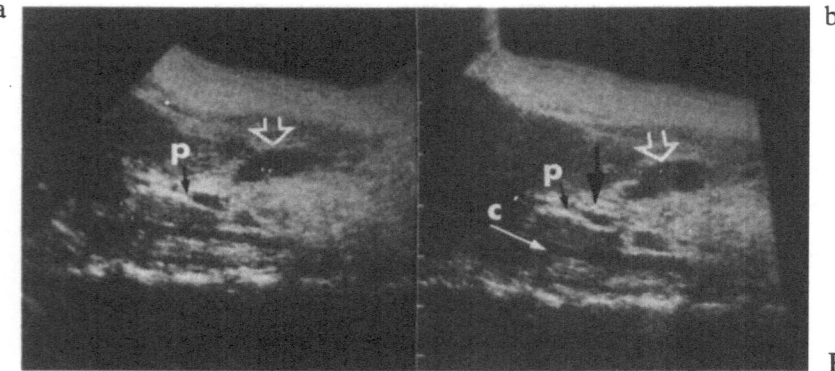

Fig. 6.2

Well...?

...The vena cava is no longer in relation with the vertebral plane. It passes through a perivascular cuff (↓ below).

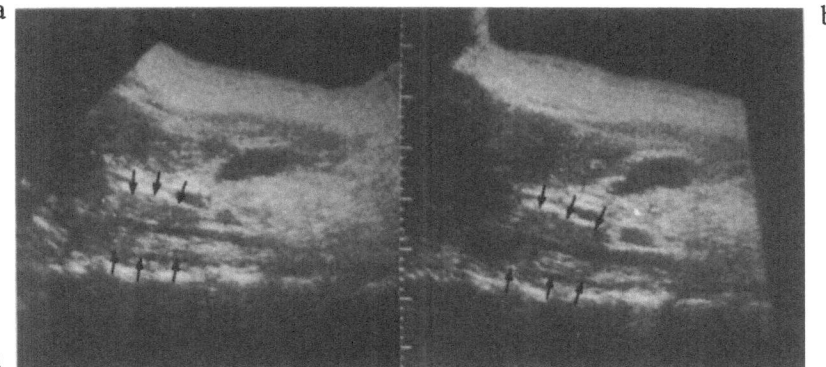

Fig. 6.2

Only adenopathies (and in rare cases, a retroperitoneal fibrosis) produce such cuff-like images. Usually, these cuffs also extend around the aorta. In this case, only the pericaval cuff is observed. There is no other ganglionic image or associated splenomegaly. There is also no ascites as might be expected since...

...since the gall bladder wall is thick (↓ below).

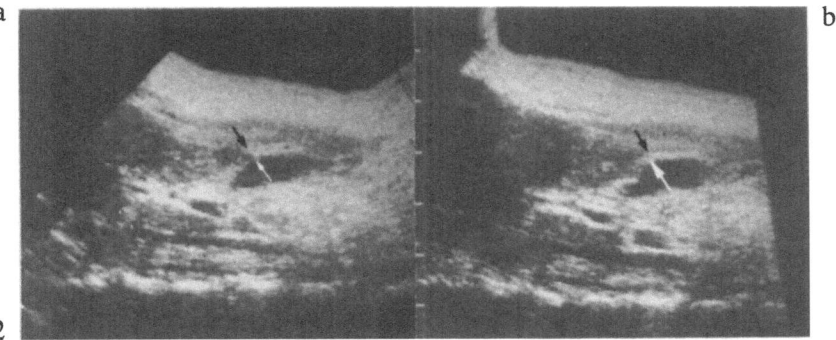

Fig. 6.2

The frozen appearance of the vena cava, which no longer shows any respiratory movement, is striking in real time.
Lymphomatous ganglionic tissue is usually sonolucent, almost liquid-like. So in this case we may wonder if the adenopathies are of some other kind. The pelvic area is examined for an ovarian lesion but appears normal.

What's to be done to advance the diagnosis?

1. First, CT for a complete evaluation of the retroperitoneal compartment and pelvic cavity.
2. Guided puncture, or failing that, surgical biopsy.

The final diagnosis in this case was lymphoma.

6.3. Mr. Poplar's clinical problems are not very specific.

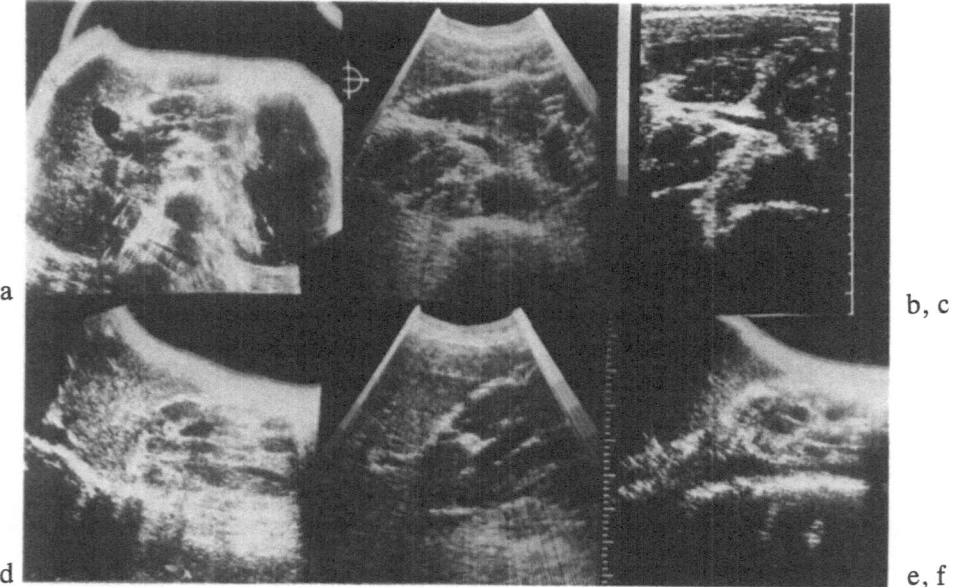

a

b, c

d

e, f

Fig. 6.3. a–c Transverse sections, **d, f** sagittal sections, **e** intercostal section

However, there is at least one clinical feature to point the way, which you will deduce immediately if you examine the transverse section 6.3a. Obviously, the spleen is enlarged and must be palpable. The sagittal coronal splenic enlargement is distinct. You have noted the less echogenic texture of the spleen compared to the liver tissue. The two kidneys are normal in appearance. Numerous nodular elements (black arrows, below) occupy the space between the large vessels, liver, and gall bladder on one side and, the spleen on the other.

They correspond to?

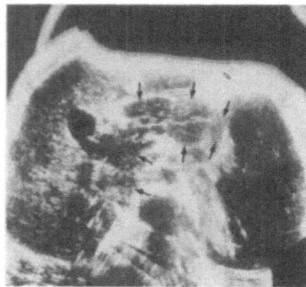

Fig. 6.3a

...Obviously, to adenopathies. Where are they situated? Are they in the retroperitoneal compartment?

We shall attempt to clarify this now. Look at Fig. 6.3b, c, below.

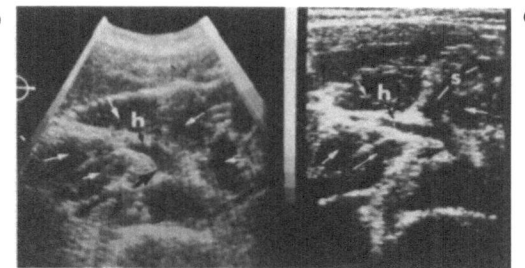

Fig. 6.3

These are epigastric sections in real time. Section 6.3b was carried out with the aid of a sector scanner, and section 6.3c with a linear array. In these almost identical sections we can identify the coeliac trunk (black arrow) and the hepatic *(h)* and splenic *(S)* arteries. This vascular network is entirely surrounded by adenopathies (white arrows). Those situated around the splenic artery are retroperitoneal. The others surround the portal vein. They are therefore within the hepatoduodenal ligament, which constitutes the right limit of the lesser omentum and contains the portal vein, hepatic artery, and bile duct. The lesser omentum, along with the stomach and gastrocolic ligament form the anterior limit of the lesser omental sac. Now look at the parasagittal section 6.3d (below). The multinodular ganglionic mass appears below the liver (large arrows).

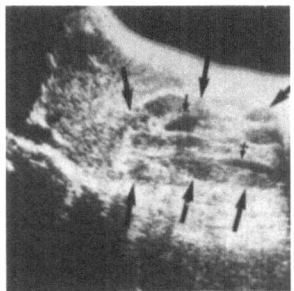

Fig. 6.3d

The superior mesenteric artery (small arrow) has been separated from its satellite vein (crossed arrow). Both penetrate and center the ganglionic mass (black arrows).

Parallel sections 6.3e, f (below) aid in the study of vascular relationships to the mass. Section 6.3e shows the superior mesenteric vein (large arrow) and vena cava (small arrows) to be quite flattened; section 6.3f shows that the aorta is also slightly compressed.

e 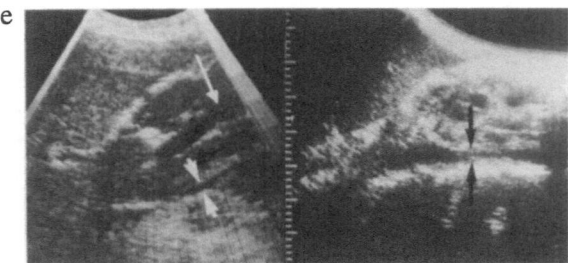 f

Fig. 6.3

These adenopathies which the mesenteric vessels center are not retroperitoneal but intramesenteric. Now look again at section 6.3a (below)

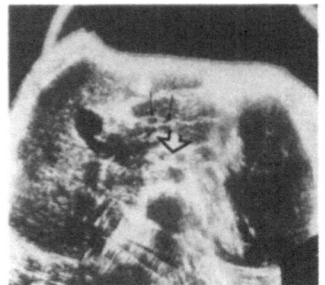 Fig. 6.3a 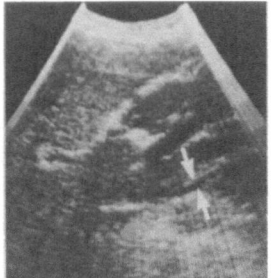 Fig. 6.3e

What do the small rounded preaortic elements indicated by an open arrow (above) correspond to?

They cannot be the mesenteric vessels, since the latter are more anterior, situated within the ganglionic mass. They are therefore two small retroperitoneal adenopathies. (Roots of the thoracic duct can also be considered.) The two mesenteric vessels (↓), surrounded by adenopathies, form Mueller's "sandwich image".

Now look at section 6.3e. Locate the laminated vena cava (↓ above).

Try to find it in a transverse section (Fig. 6.3a, b, or c, p. 66).

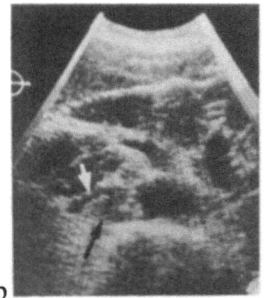 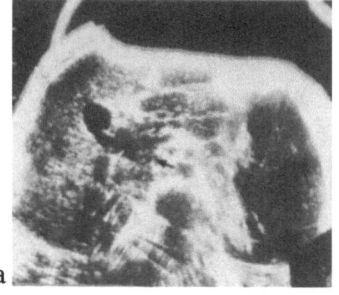

Fig. 6.3b   Fig. 6.3a

The vessel is indicated by a white arrow in Fig. 6.3b above.

It is completely flattened and forced forward by a retrovenous adenopathy (black arrow above). In section 6.3a the adenopathy is also seen posterior to the vena cava ($\downarrow$).

Can you locate this adenopathy in a sagittal section (Fig. 6.3d, p. 67)? It is indicated by black arrows in section 6.3d, below.

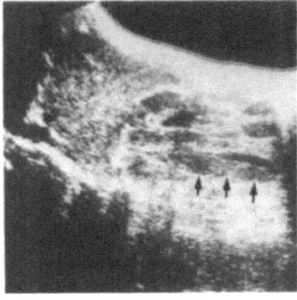 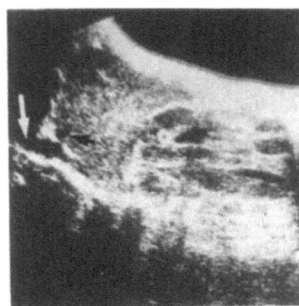

Fig. 6.3d   Fig. 6.3d

One last question: What does the fluid area indicated by a white arrow in Fig. 6.3d (above) correspond to?

This is not a pleural effusion, but a normal image of the junction between inferior vena cava and right atrium. This is confirmed by the image of the extremity of the medial hepatic vein (black arrow), laterally sectioned near its junction with the vena cava.

The splenic and ganglionic images are typical of lymphoma. Apart from a chest X-ray, should other procedures be carried out? In this particular case, exploration of abdominal ganglia by lymphography is unnecessary. Anyway, lymphography is unlikely to show mesenteric adenopathies. However, it may be useful for the pelvic area. Since CT is recommended in the mediastinal evaluation of lymphoma, a few pelvic CT scans may be performed as a complement to the thoracic examination. Ultrasonic evaluation is sufficient for the abdomen itself.

Chapter 7

Postoperative Complications

7.1. and 7.2. Mrs. Birch and Mrs. Cottonwood underwent digestive surgery one week ago. Both have fever; both are in pain.

7.1. Mrs. Birch had a cholecystectomy; in her case, a puriform fluid flows from the opening to the Kehr drain, which transports clear bile.

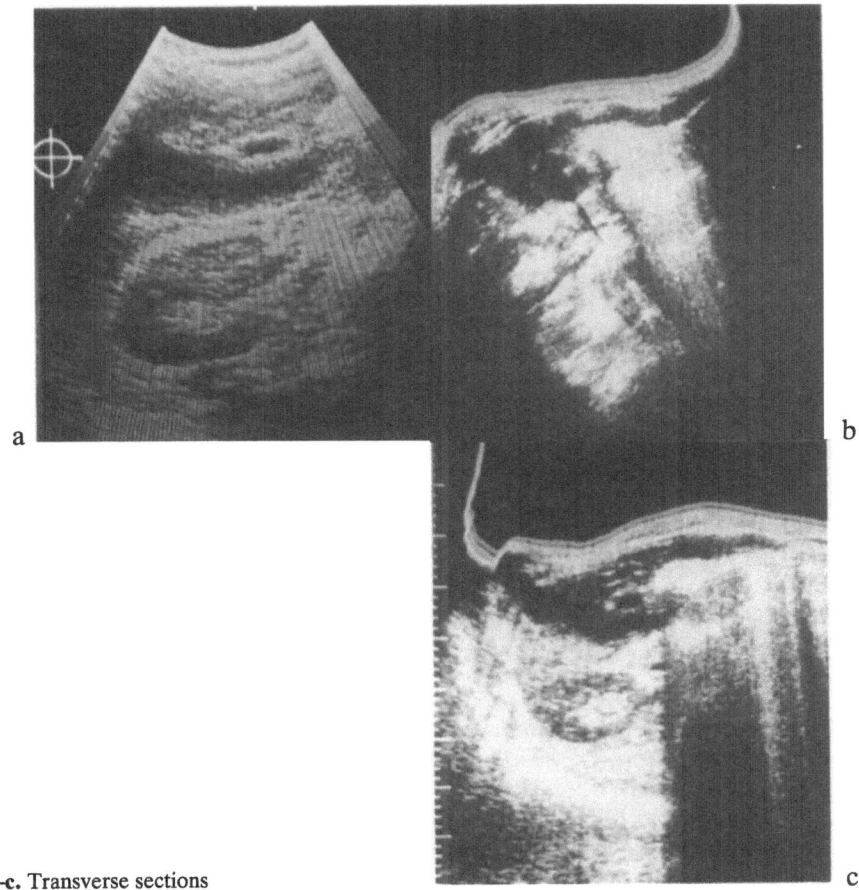

Fig. 7.1a–c. Transverse sections

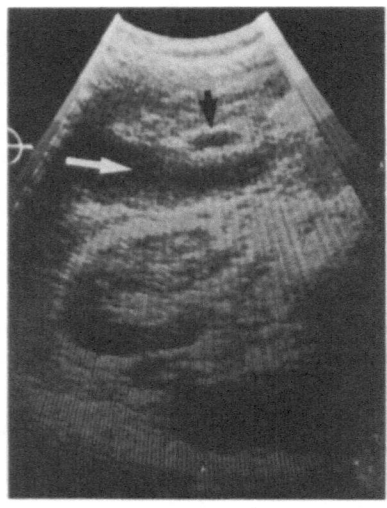

Fig. 7.1a

A transverse section (Fig. 7.1a) shows a collection near the liver (white arrow, above) and kidney. The collection doesn't enter Morison's pouch, which remains virtual. Which important anatomical relationship allows us to locate this collection?

The answer is the transverse section of the portal vein (black arrow, above). It runs with its satellites (common bile duct and hepatic artery) within the hepatoduodenal ligament which represents, as you will remember, the anterior limit of the foramen of Winslow.

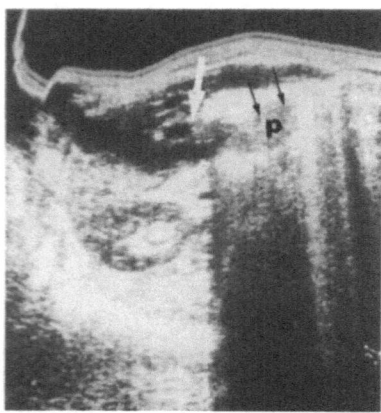

Fig. 7.1c

The hepatoduodenal ligament can also be seen in section 7.1c (white arrow, above). Note, lateral to the external wall of the portal vein, the thin section of the common bile duct. The section of the hepatic artery is displayed just below the tip of the white arrowhead. If you follow the collection to the left, you will see the fine line (black arrows) which marks the posterior wall of the stomach, anterior to the pancreas *(p)*.

Thus, you will have located the lesser omental sac itself, which remains virtual – perhaps temporarily in this case. The abscess is working its way outwards by another route. In Fig. 7.1b below you can see it penetrating the abdominal wall (arrow).

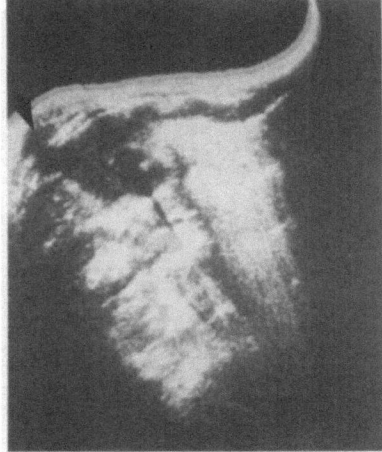

Fig. 7.1b

Figure 7.1c below shows an opening in the abdominal wall, reaching the skin, which bulges (arrow).

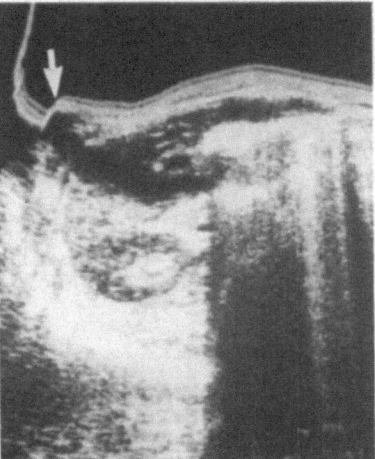

Fig. 7.1c

Evidently we are seeing a subhepatic abscess ready to externalize itself and threatening to reach the lesser omental sac.

Everything will be sorted out within the hour, with a good slice of the scalpel. There is about half a liter of pus. It would also have been possible to install a double catheter under ultrasonic guidance to drain and wash the cavity, in which case surgery could have been avoided.

7.2. Mrs. Cottonwood is 72 but young in spirit. She underwent emergency surgery for acute appendicitis. A week later, the surgeon drained an abscess of the right iliac fossa. Several days later fever started again. There is no particularly painful area. Is it a recurrence of the earlier abscess or another suppuration?

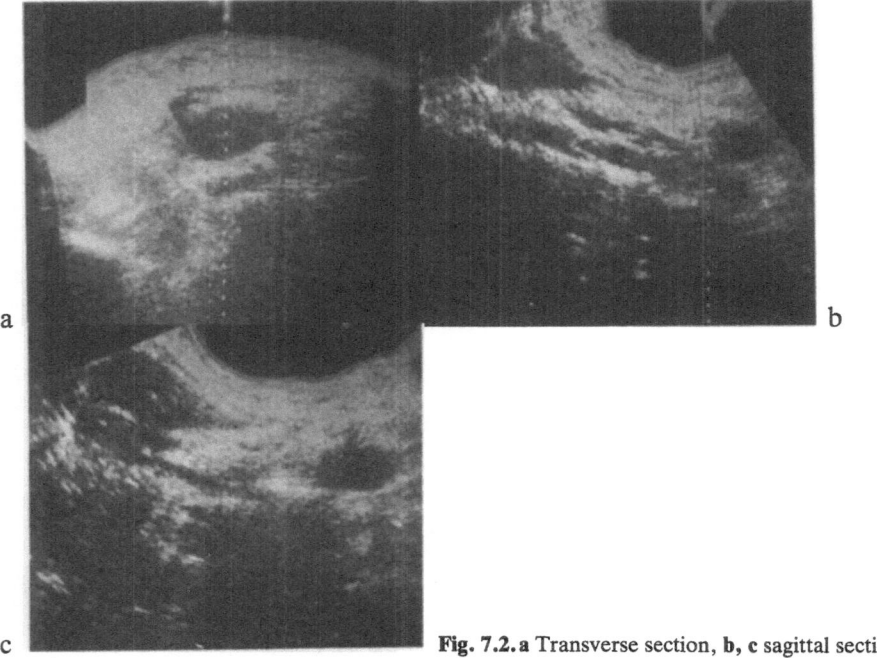

a

b

c   **Fig. 7.2. a** Transverse section, **b, c** sagittal sections

Sections of the right iliac fossa show no collection. On the other hand a global transverse section (Fig. 7.2a) shows a distinct collection (arrows, below) at the level of the umbilicus (indicated by the centimeter scale).

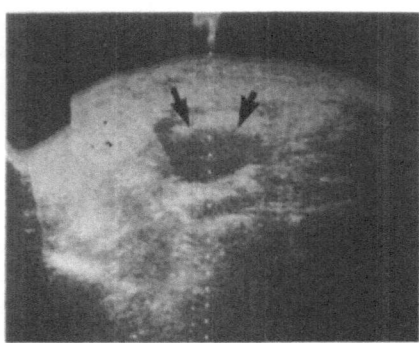

Fig. 7.2a

74

A sagittal section (Fig. 7.2b) through the aorta *(a)* and SMV *(V)* also shows this collection (arrow, below).

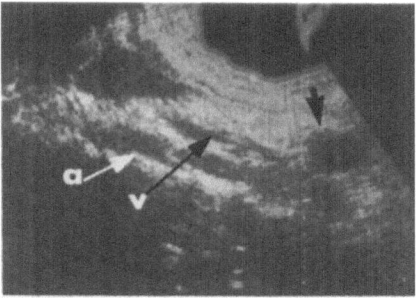

Fig. 7.2b

Good. The abscess is found. Can we indicate its position to the surgeon with greater precision?

Yes. The superior mesenteric vein allows us to locate the mesentery; in addition, a transonic band (arrow, below) runs posterior to an echogenic strip and anterior to the collection (Fig. 7.2a, b).

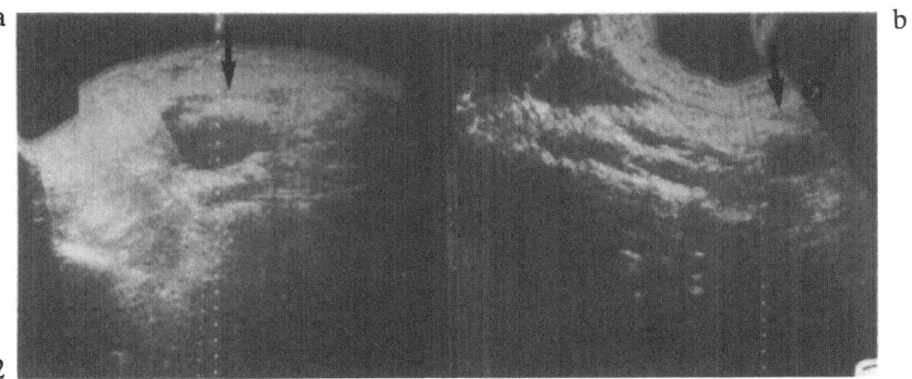

Fig. 7.2

This echogenic strip corresponds to the greater omentum. Therefore, we can state that the collection is deep, situated between greater omentum and intestinal loops. This is an area which is usually rather difficult to explore with sonography, due to the masking effect of intestinal gas.

So, when possible, it is useful to have patients, in whom postoperative suppuration is suspected, undergo a CT scan, which may show deeper infections with greater precision.

But we have just demonstrated once again that a thorough ultrasound analysis will often identify peritoneal and retroperitoneal structures with great precision.

7.3. Mr. Cherry has had a cholecystectomy. He also complains of pain in the right side and has fever.

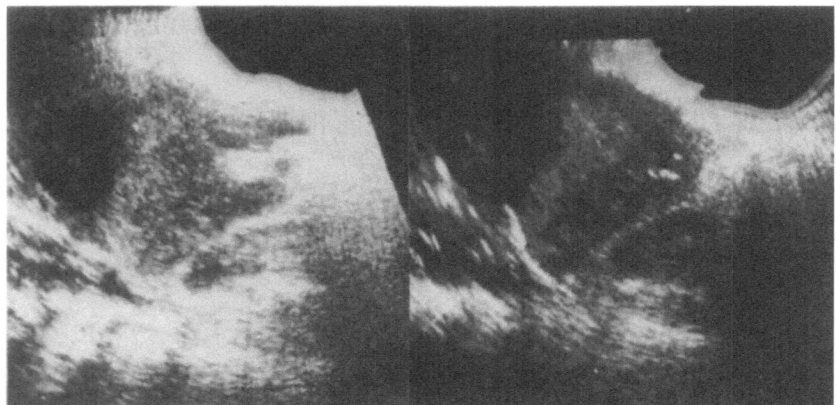

a   b

Fig. 7.3

The sonograms in Fig. 7.3 are sagittal sections of the right upper quadrant. Here you will have noticed a large collection (white arrows, below) between the liver and the diaphragm. It's a subphrenic abscess.

Should we close the case?

No. There's still something to see ... (answer[1] at bottom of page).

a   b

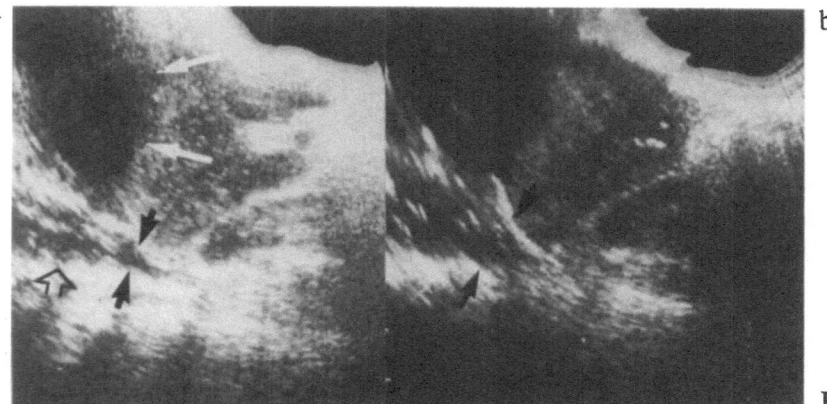

Fig. 7.3

---

1 There is a right pleural effusion (black arrows, above), since a sonolucent supradiaphragmatic area is displayed. The posterior thoracic wall (open arrow), which is not normally shown owing to interruption of the ultrasound by pulmonary air, is visible here

7.4. and 7.5. Mrs. Cypress and Mrs. Peach both had surgery several years ago. They both complain of distension.

7.4. Mrs. Cypress had a left colectomy for colonic cancer.

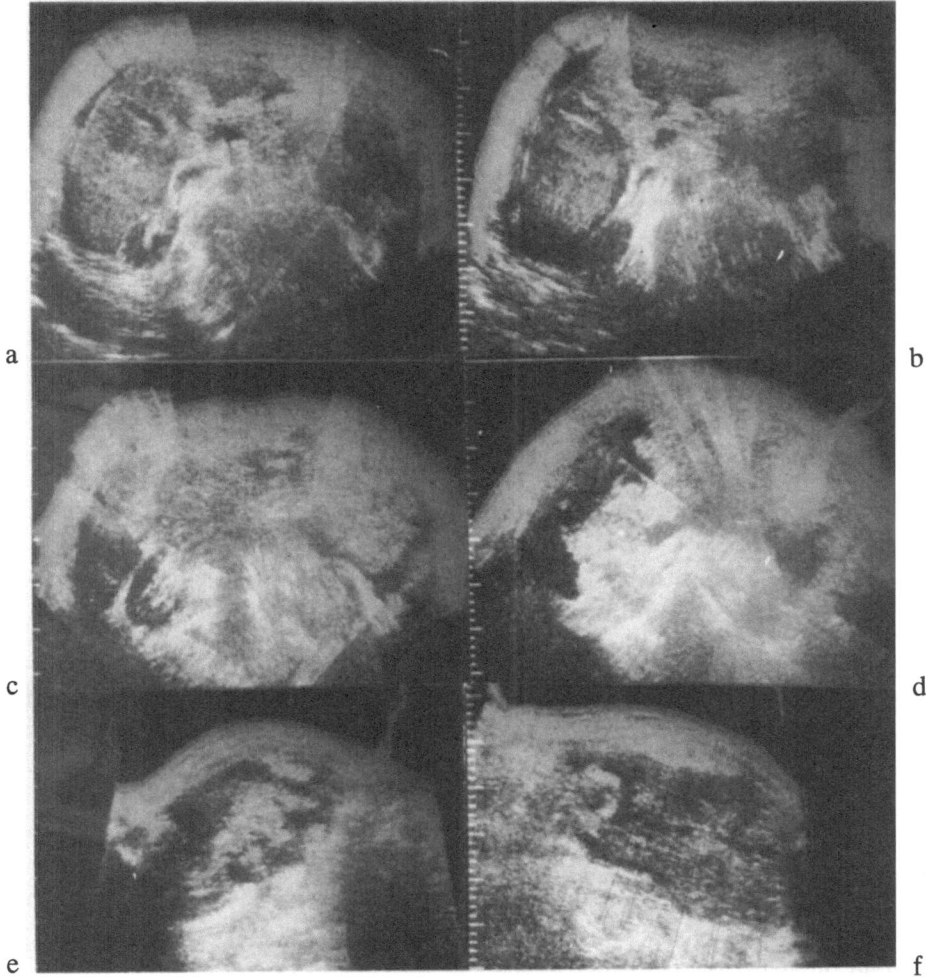

a

b

c

d

e

f

Fig. 7.4. a–e Transverse sections, **f** sagittal section

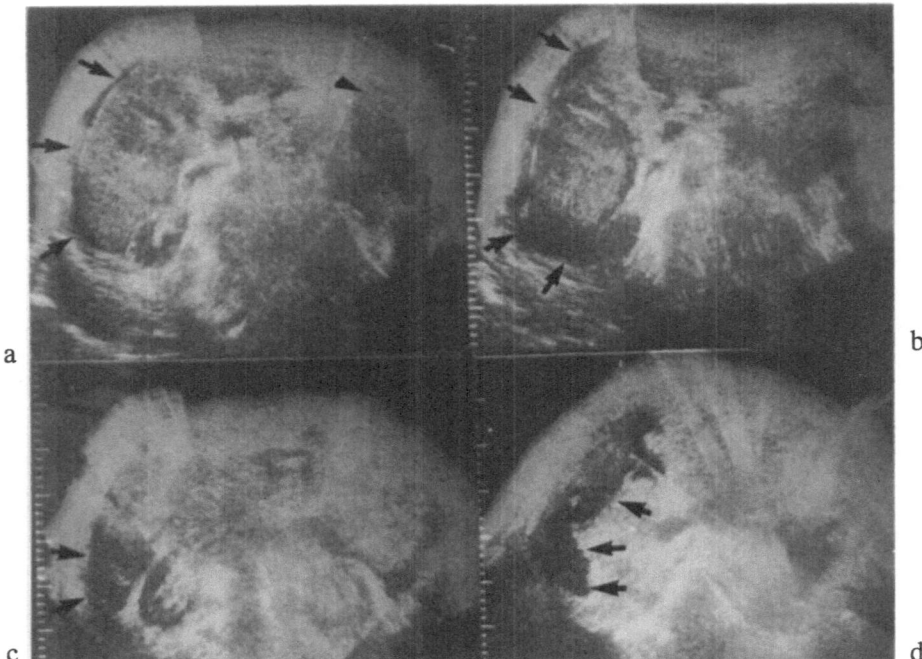

Fig. 7.4

Free ascites is clearly seen in the four transverse sections 7.4a–d. A sonotranspa-rent band, typical of a fluid effusion, is present around the liver (↓ above).

Compare this image of perihepatic fluid to that of pleural effusion in Fig. 1.1a, b. Small quantities of intraperitoneal fluid are shown in pre- and laterohepatic sites, whereas the pleural effusion is retrohepatic. Why is there usually no retrohepatic peritoneal effusion? (Answer[1] at bottom of page.)

Now we will analyse the different peritoneal recesses.

Is there liquid in the lesser omental sac?

No. Stomach and pancreas are in direct contact (Fig. 7.4a next page). There is fluid, however, in Morison's pouch (arrows, Fig. 7.4a, next page).

---

1 Because of the presence of the trangular ligament

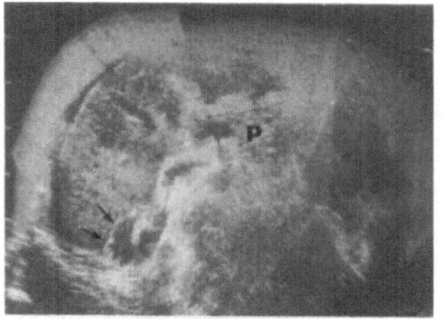

Fig. 7.4a

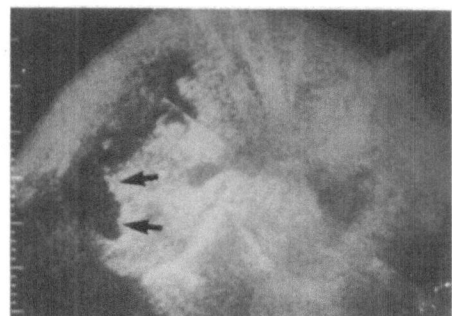

Fig. 7.4d

Section 7.4d shows fluid in the right paracolic gutter (arrows, above).

Sections 7.4e, f are of the right iliac fossa. Here is a mass with ill-defined contours (arrows, below) containing several liquid zones.

Do they correspond to free or septated ascites?

e 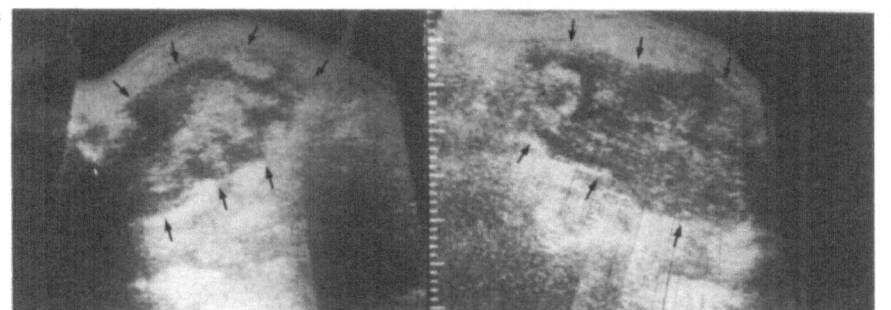 f

Fig. 7.4

The answer is given to the sonologist on the spot by a positional change of the patient to left lateral decubitus. The image does not change. It therefore corresponds to septated ascites containing fixed intestinal loops. This type of image is often found in metastatic peritoneal carcinomatosis; it is also encountered in pseudomyxoma peritonei (and in tuberculous ascites). We can now attempt to confirm this diagnosis with a cytological study following guided puncture. Gastrointestinal series and a enema are indispensable to decide whether a preventive surgical derivation is called for, if occlusion threatens.

7.5. Mrs. Peach was operated on and irradiated for ovarian cancer 5 years ago. Now her abdomen is distended. Palpation reveals nothing very particular.

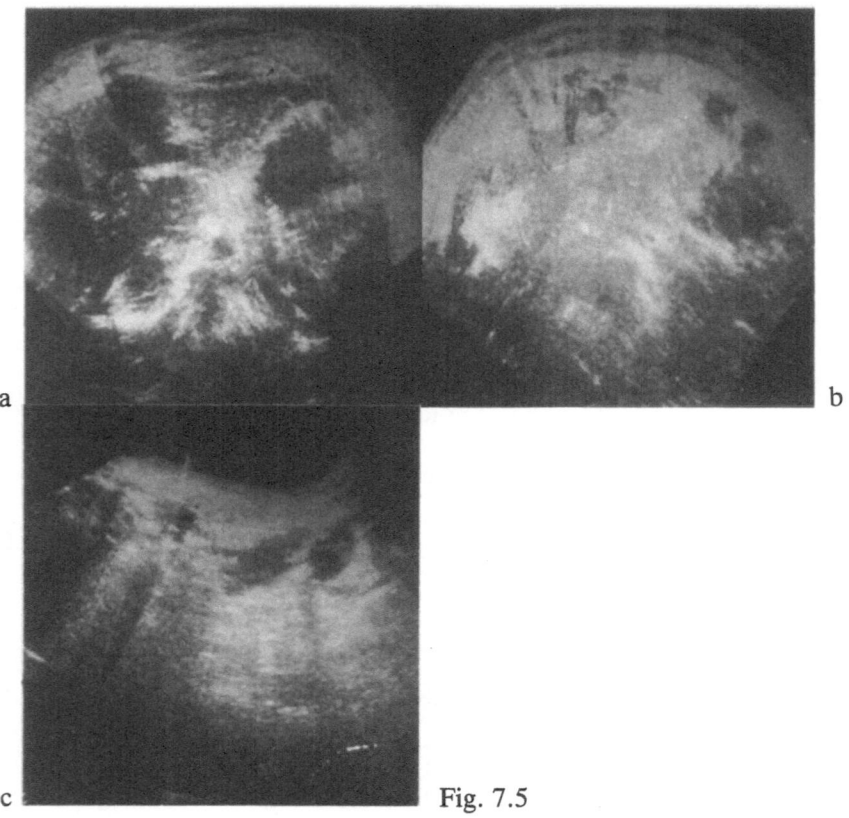

a

b

c

Fig. 7.5

Figures 7.5a, b are parallel transverse sections, one taken at the xyphoid level and the other at the level of the umbilicus. Figure 7.5c is a sagittal section of the left flank.

A restricted mass is found in the left upper quadrant (↓ below), near the left hepatic lobe. It has no distinct relationship with organs other then intestinal loops.

a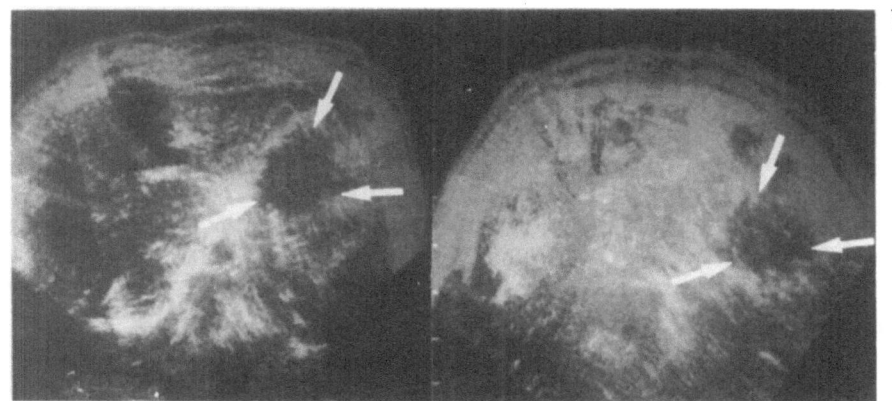b

Fig. 7.5

This image closely resembles that which we have just seen in the iliac fossa of Mrs. Cypress (Fig. 7.4e, f, p. 79). It is highly suggestive of peritoneal deposits. However, it is not possible to differentiate metastatic nodules, areas of septated ascites, and neighboring fixed intestinal loops which may themselves be distended and filled with fluid.

Is there also free ascites?

Yes. A small liquid strip (black arrow, Fig. 7.5a, below) is seen directly in front of the liver. In that area, peritoneal deposits have a similar pattern. Differentiation is obtained by positional studies.

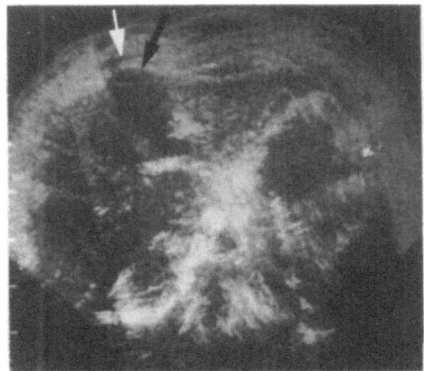

Fig. 7.5a

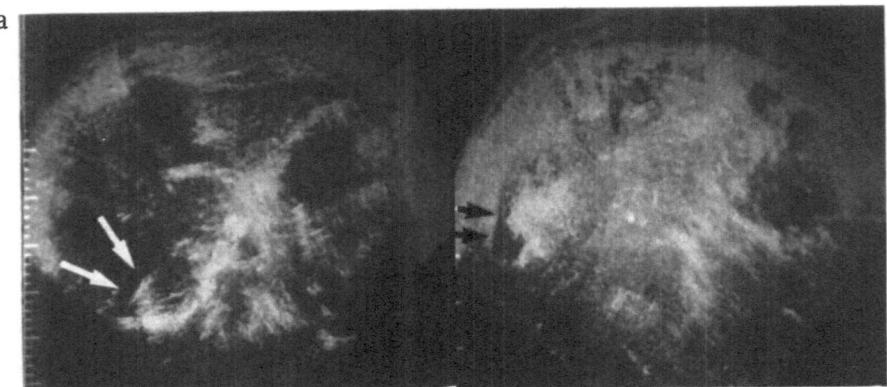

Fig. 7.5

A neighboring intraparietal fatty strip (white arrow) should not be confused with this thin ascitic band. A small amount of liquid is also found in Morison's pouch (↓ Fig. 7.5a, above), as well as in the right paracolic gutter (↓ Fig. 7.5b, above).

If there is any doubt between fluid and fatty strip (only fat rich in connective fibers, e.g. perirenal fat, is echogenic), any image variations during the respiratory cycle and positional changes should be particularly scrutinized: fatty patterns remain constant but free fluid collections do not.

What does the lowest oval sonolucent image in the sagittal section of Fig. 7.5c below correspond to? (p. 80).

It is the left lateral part of the bladder (black arrow, below).

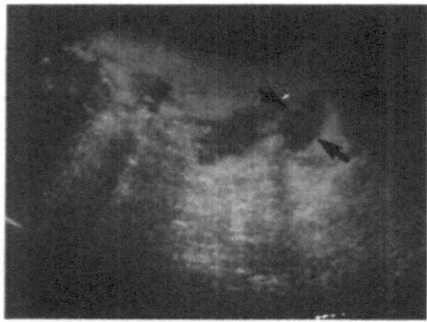

Fig. 7.5c

What can still be done to clarify the diagnosis?

- First, CT. In this particular case CT showed that the left mass mainly corresponded to septated ascites.
- Possibly, guided fine-needle puncture for a cytologic study. This procedure is only useful if the origin of the malignant ascites is unknown. Here, thanks to the clinical history, it can logically be attributed to the ovarian tumor.
- Conventional X-ray studies of the digestive tract may be justified in order to consider the possibility of palliative derivation.

7.6. Mrs. Tulip had a left colectomy 3 years ago. She complains of pain in the left upper quadrant.

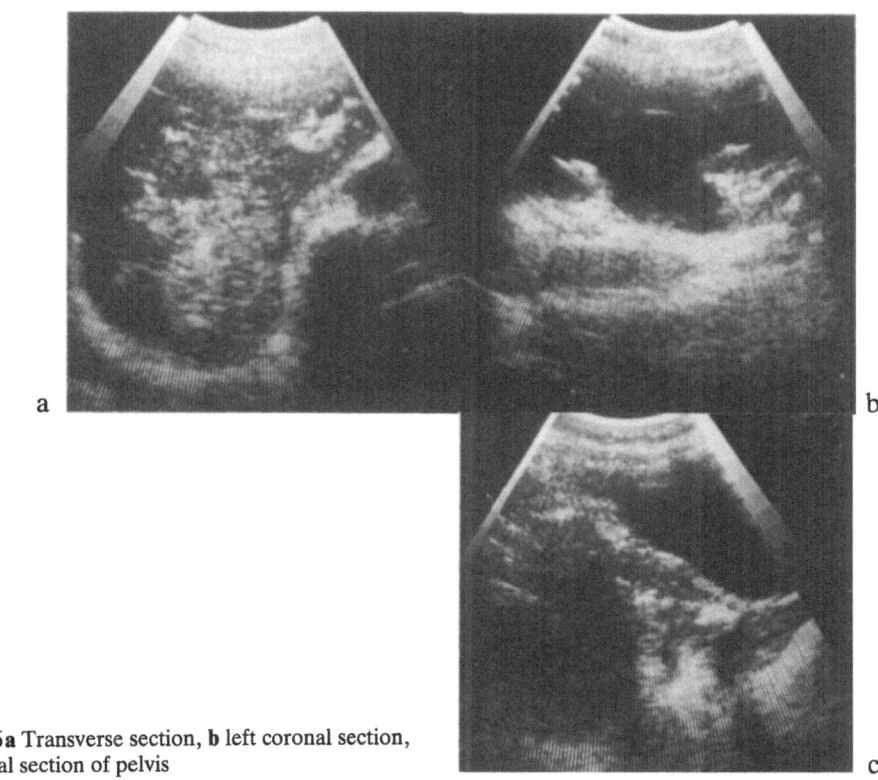

a

b

Fig. 7.6a Transverse section, **b** left coronal section, **c** sagittal section of pelvis

c

You have certainly recognized the presence of hepatic metastases in the transverse hepatic section (Fig. 7.6a, ↓ below).

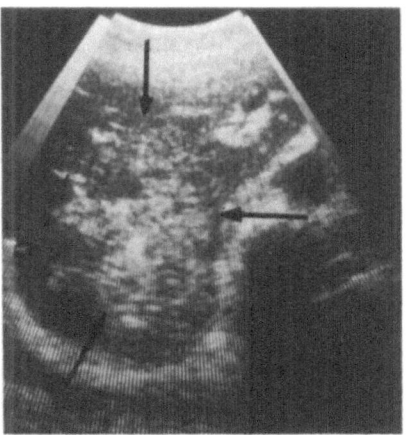

Fig. 7.6a

This association of echogenic areas and transonic nodules could, strictly speaking, suggest an alveolar echinococcosis in some countries. However, the common clinical history of this rare parasitosis (professional risk[1] in particular) is absent, whereas carcinological antecedents are obvious. Chronic active hepatitis and hepatoma are other diagnostic possibilites which may require guided puncture, after multiple hemangiomas have been ruled out by contrast-enhanced CT.

The coronal section carried out by left lateral approach shows dilatation of the entire renal collecting system (Fig. 7.6b, below): dilated calices(h), renal pelvis (open arrow), and ureter (black arrow) are displayed.

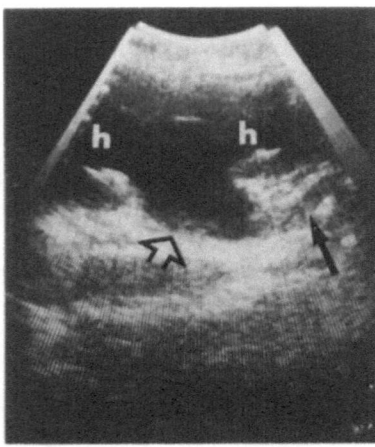

Fig. 7.6b

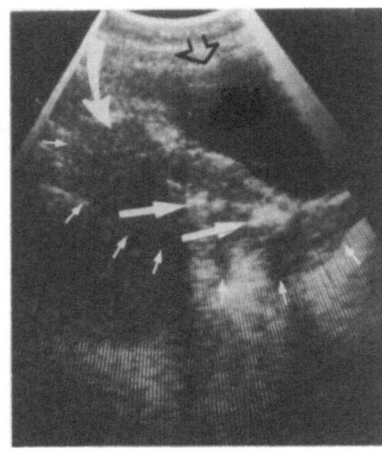

Fig. 7.6c

We continue the exploration by examining the pelvis (Fig. 7.6c, above). The uterus (Fig. 7.6c, small arrows, above) is fibromatous. The main fibromatous nodule (curved arrow) is partially masked by a diffractive shadow (due to sound-bending). The open arrow points to the bladder, the large arrows to calcified foci.

Finally the left hydronephrosis was not due to ureteric compression arising from the enlarged uterus, but to a pelvic carcinomatosis related to the colonic carcinoma.

---

1 outdoor work such as farming, lumber-cutting, etc.

Chapter 8

The Yellow Peril

Patients Sweetgum, Persimmon, Palm, Sassafras, and Chestnut all have something in common: heavy or thin, tall or small, bald or hairy, they all have the complexion of a (slightly faded) buttercup.

8.1. Mr. Sweetgum.

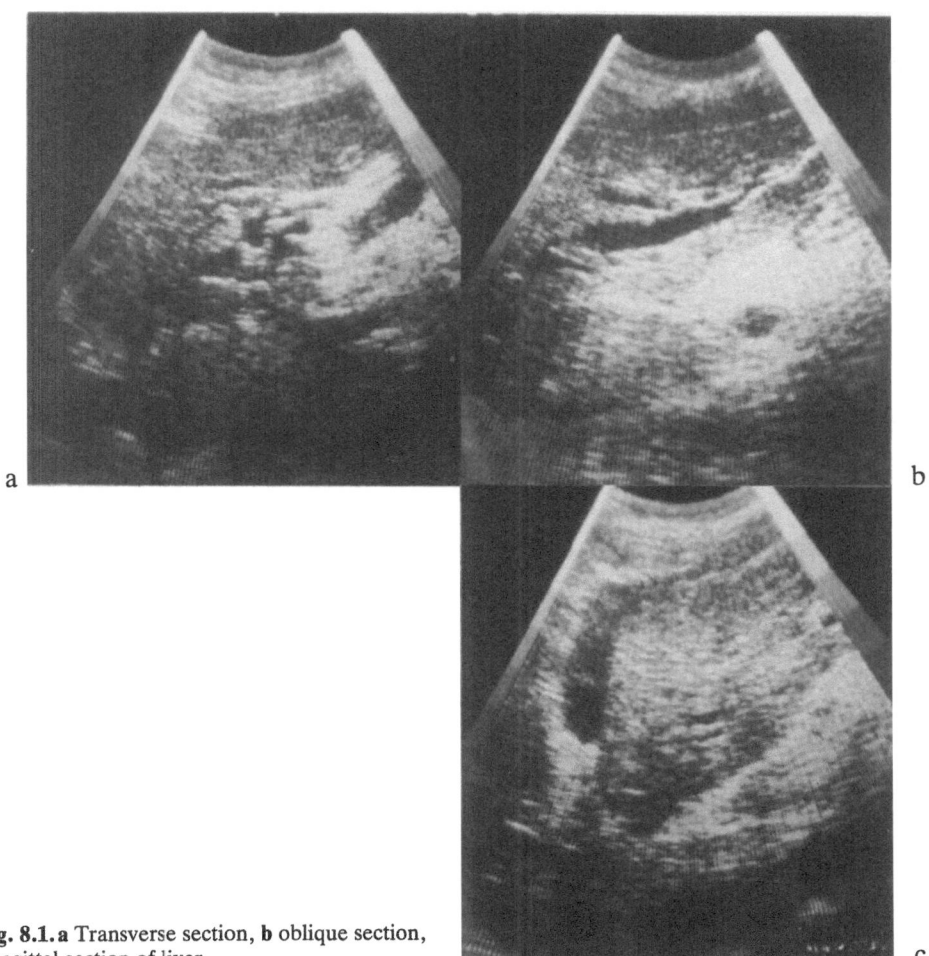

a

b

c

Fig. 8.1. a Transverse section, **b** oblique section, **c** sagittal section of liver

a) Does Mr. Sweetgum have signs of biliary obstruction?

Yes: Fig. 8.1a below...

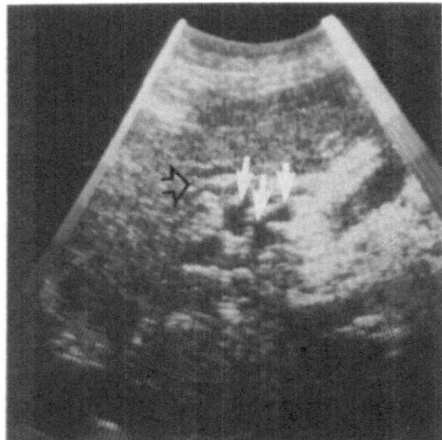
Fig. 8.1a

...shows an unusual intrahepatic ductal network ($\downarrow$) and an intrahepatic gun sign (open arrow).

An intrahepatic gun sign is also seen in the sagittal section of the left lobe in Fig. 8.1c (open arrow, below).

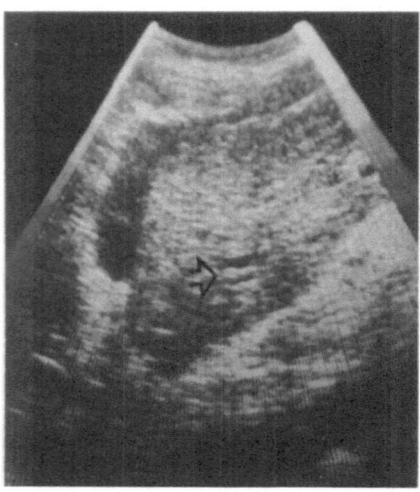
Fig. 8.1c

Thus, dilatation of the bile ducts is a first obvious conclusion.

b) At what level is the obstruction?

A subcostal oblique section (Fig. 8.1b, below) ...

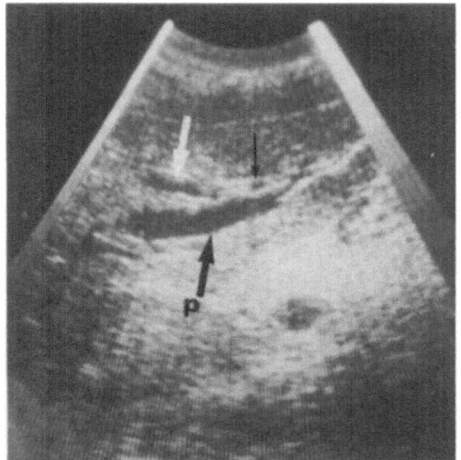

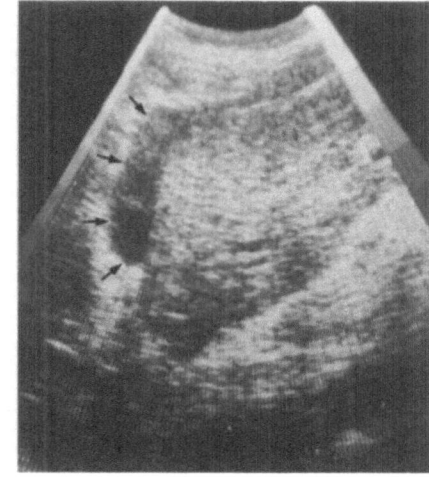

Fig. 8.1b   Fig. 8.1c

...shows the portal vein *(p)*. The prevenous ductal structure (white arrow) cannot correspond to the bile duct since it is separated from the portal vein. Epigastric scanning in real time confirms that it is the hepatic artery. The common bile duct is seen more caudally (black arrow). Its diameter is normal. Thus, the obstruction is hilar.
There is no tumoral mass at the level of the hilum. We are therefore probably dealing with a primary biliary carcinoma, infiltrating the biliary confluence.

Before considering the next step, there is one more abnormality to find. You'll find it (if you have not already done so) in sagittal section 8.1c. There is ascites between the liver and diaphram (↓ above), with all the suspicions and problems that entails.

This ascites had not been clinically recognized.
In this patient, we will puncture the ascites for a cytological study. A percutaneous cholangiography should then be carried out to confirm the diagnosis of hilar obstruction before performing a palliative internal drainage: hilar obstruction constitutes one of the precise and restrictive indications for percutaneous cholangiography.

8.2. Mrs. Persimmon has jaudice without accompanying clinical symptoms.

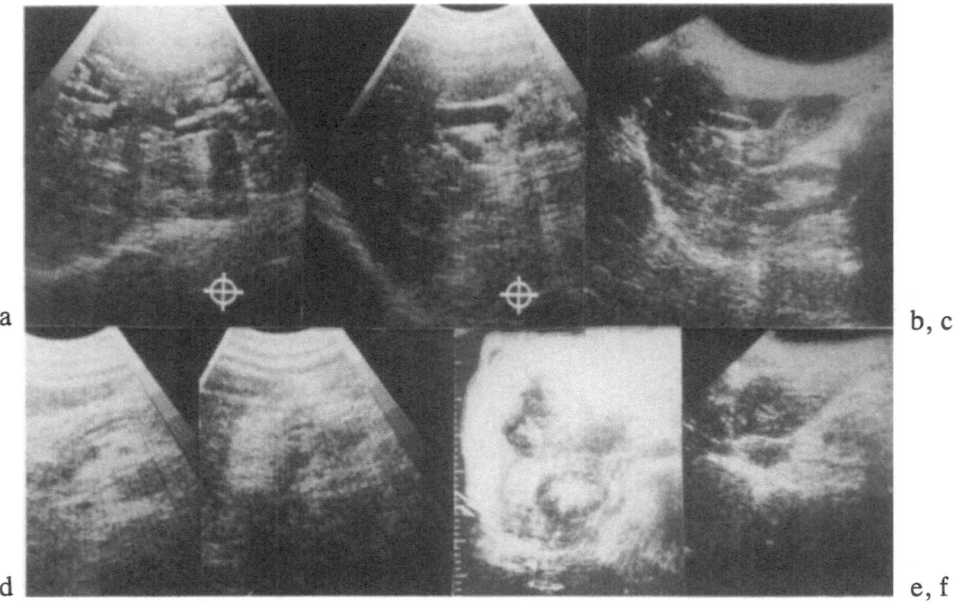

a   b, c

d   e, f

Fig. 8.2. a Intercostal section, **b, c, e, g** sagittal sections, **f** transverse section

Intercostal section 8.2a (above, then below) shows a hepatic biliary network which is highly dilated ($\downarrow$). It also shows a hilar gun sign.

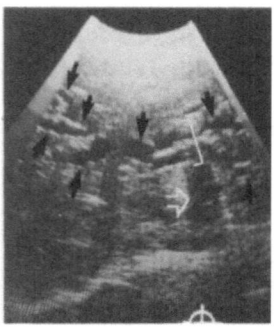   Fig. 8.2a

An acoustic shadow (open arrow) is observed – posterior to the portal vein. This shadow is probably the result of diffraction at the level of a ductal bend. Conversely, there are areas of increased acoustic transmission behind several bile ducts. This phenomenon is due to lesser attenuation within bile than within blood.

Sagittal section 8.2b shows a subhepatic gun sign (p. 88, then below, open arrow).

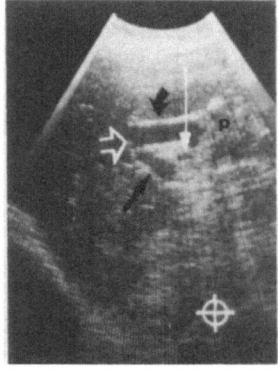

Fig. 8.2b

It is possible to recognize the subhepatic topography of this double image thanks to ...?

...the round section of a small interductal element, which corresponds to the right branch of the hepatic artery (white arrow, above). This arterial branch runs between the bile duct (curved arrow) and portal vein (black arrow). The bile duct's relation to the pancreas *(p)* is displayed more caudally. The pancreas appears normal in this section.

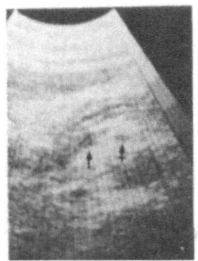 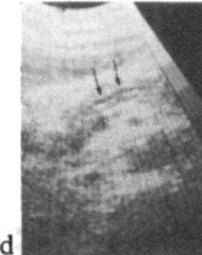 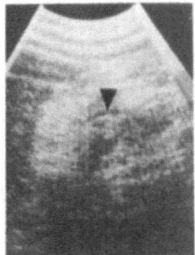

Fig. 8.2 d   d   e

Now look at transverse section 8.2d (p. 88, then above). It shows the pancreas, anterior to the eyeglass image of the mesenteric vessels. The vein is the ductal element situated ... farthest to the right? or to the left?

... Farthest to the right (↓). At this level the vascular sections are more than 1 cm apart, since this is the area where the mesenteric vein curves to the right to join the splenoportal confluence. The venous lumen is slightly larger and more transparent than the arterial lumen, whereas the venous wall is thinner. Thus, the left vascular juxta-aortic element (crossed arrow) corresponds to the superior mesenteric artery.

A major abnormality in this section is...?

...dilatation of the pancreatic duct (arrows, Fig. 8.2d, e, above).

The binomial "dilatation of the pancreatic duct + dilatation of the common bile duct" confirms obstruction of the ampulla by a pancreatic tumor or ampulloma. Interpretation of this binomial is essential when the tumor is too small to be clearly outlined. In this case, the tumor (↓ Fig. 8.2f, g, below) is evident. It would have been recognized even without dilatation of the pancreatic duct.

f 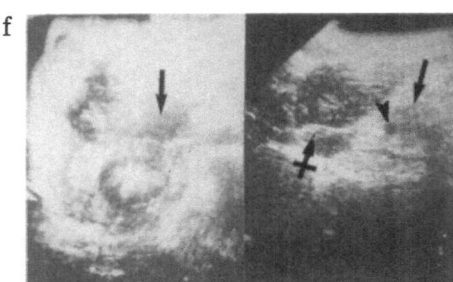 g

Fig. 8.2

We still have two anatomical questions to ask concerning Fig. 8.2g (above), which, as you remember, is a sagittal section:
a) What is the linear feature separating the caudate lobe from the right lobe of the liver? (↕)
b) What is the small rounded sonolucent element observed in contact with the superior border of the pancreas (arrowhead)?
...a) A connective tract including the obliterated remains of the ductus venosus which joins portal and caval systems during the fetal stage.
...b) A sagittal section of the splenic artery or vein (probably the artery considering the appearance of the vascular lumen).
So we are dealing with jaundice simply caused by pancreatic cancer. Remember this binomial: "Dilatation of the pancreatic duct + dilatation of the common bile duct = mass of the ampullar region".
Also note that we have not been concerned with the gall bladder, since analysis of it is less determinative than analysis of the bile duct. It should, however, always be checked as it may be lithiasic or even tumoral. With multiple sections we will verify the absence of hepatic metastases. The possibility of a false heterogeneous appearance due to intrahepatic biliary dilatations should be kept in mind.
Should any other preoperative procedures be carried out? The only one that can be considered is CT, to complete the study of the tumoral extension. Other examinations, and particularly instrumental cholangiography, would just mean added risk to the patient and his wallet (or the social security's).

90

8.3. Mrs. Palm also has jaundice.

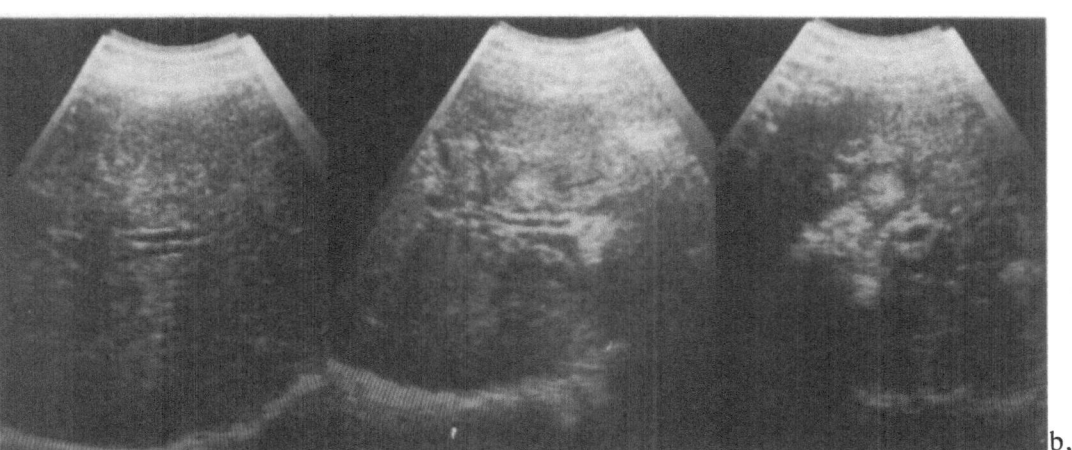

a

Fig. 8.3.a Oblique recurrent section, **b** subcostal oblique section, **c** transverse section

b, c

a) Are there objective signs of obstruction?

Yes: oblique recurrent section 8.3a shows several gun images (above, then ↓ below).

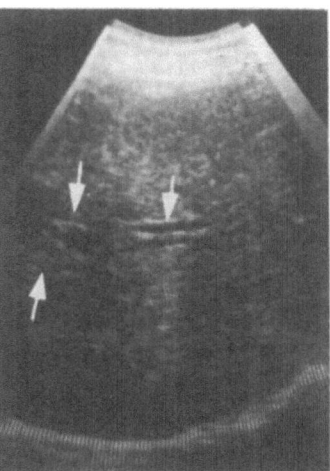

Fig. 8.3a

91

b) At what level is the obstruction?

An oblique section of the right upper quadrant (Fig. 8.3b, below) shows the hepatic duct (↓) anterior to the portal vein *(P)*. Its diameter is not more than half that of the portal vein, i.e. it is a normal value. So we can expect a hilar obstruction.

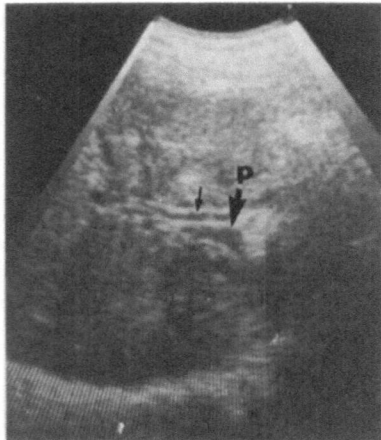

Fig. 8.3b

c) What is the nature of the obstruction?

A transverse section at the hilar level (Fig. 8.3c) shows intraparenchymal nodular lesions (↓ below).

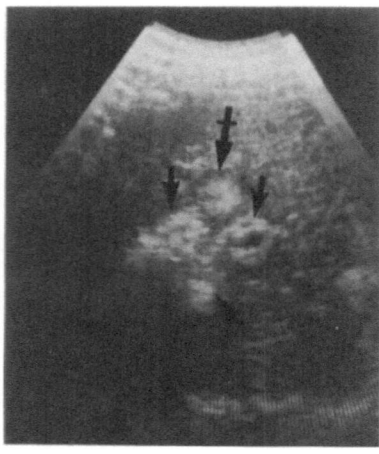

Fig. 8.3c

One of these is a bull's-eye nodule (crossed arrow). We are therefore dealing with metastases rather than with the intraparenchymal extension of a biliary carcinoma.

You have certainly already noticed several small nodules in Fig. 8.3b (p. 91, then below).

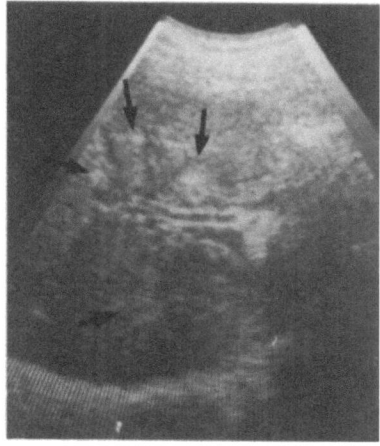

Fig. 8.3b

The primary cancer was located in the terminal colon.

Can you further analyse section 8.3c for ductal features?

See p. 91, then below. It is possible to identify the small section of the hepatic artery ($\downarrow$), and also the non-dilated common hepatic duct ($\ddagger$) anterior to the portal vein (white arrow), within the hepato-duodenal ligament.

Fig. 8.3c

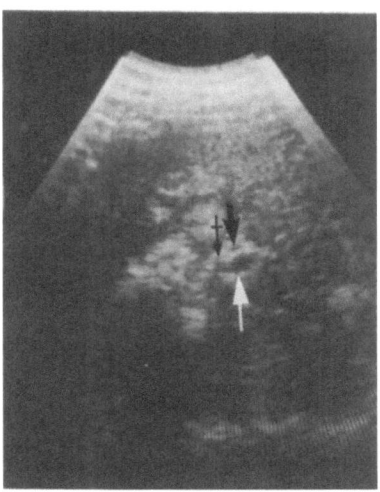

What else can be done for the patient?

Whereas instrumental cholangiography was clearly not called for in the previous case, it is essential here, primarily to attempt an internal, or failing that, an external palliative drainage.

8.4. Mrs. Sassafras. First, a riddle: what is Mrs. Sassafras' complexion like? We won't insist.

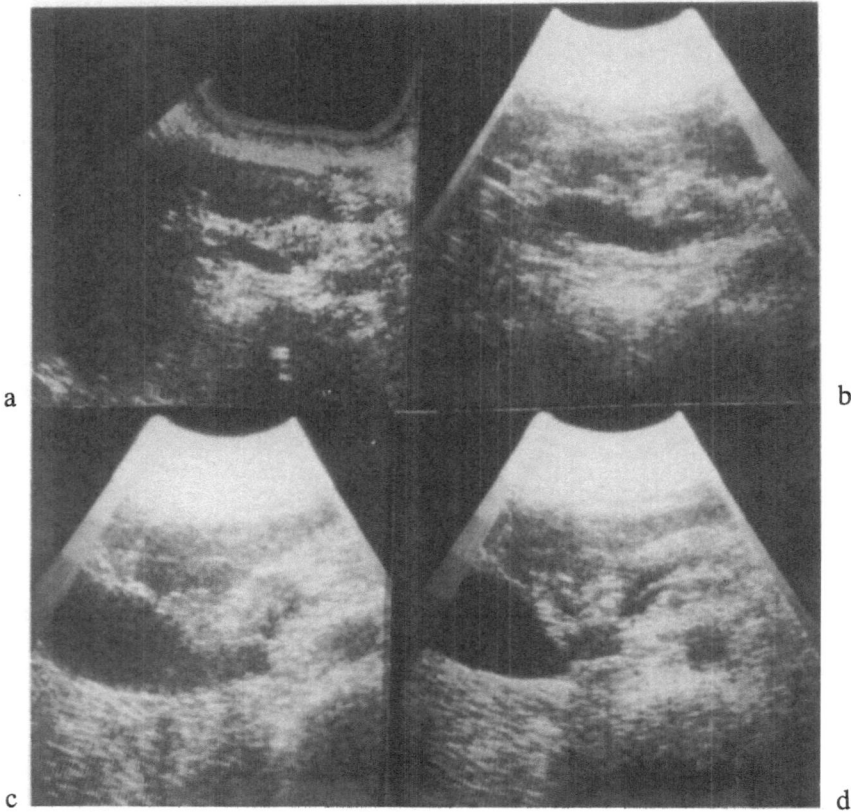

Fig. 8.4. a, b Oblique sections (right upper quadrant), **c, d** parallel transverse sections

This case is not an opportunity for us to exercise our geological knowledge: the enlarged gall bladder (↓ Fig. 8.4c, d, below) is completely free of stones.

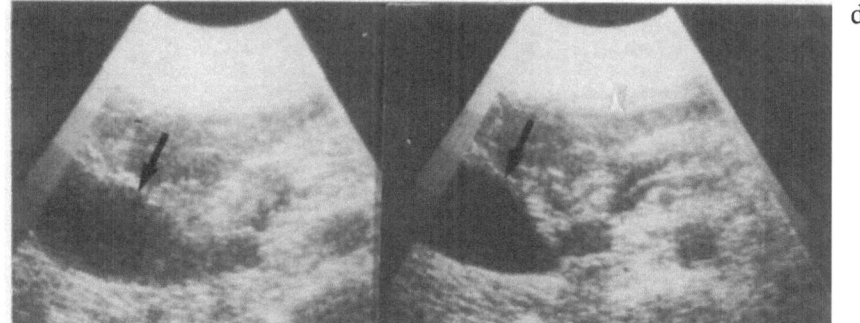

Fig. 8.4

But you should have recognized the chance to practise your mathematical expertise: here we have an example of our binomial "dilated pancreatic duct + dilated bile duct". First, the bile duct: oblique sections of the right upper quadrant show a highly dilated common bile duct (white arrows, Fig. 8.4a, b, below).

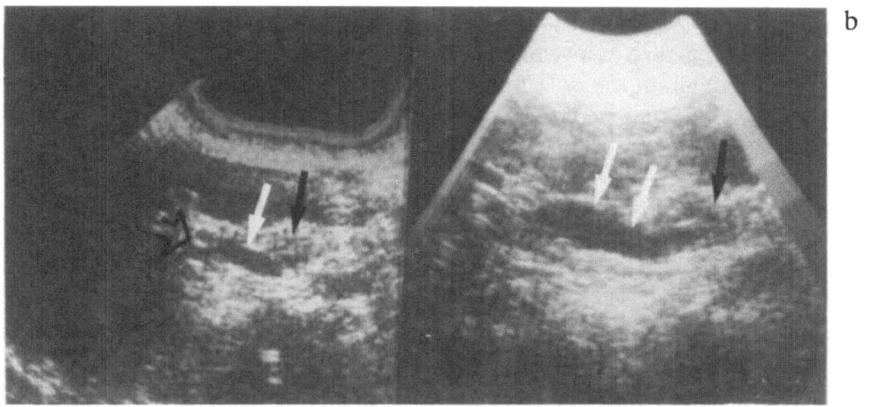

Fig. 8.4

The biliary nature of this ductal segment is confirmed (if necessary) by a subhepatic gun sign (open arrow, Fig. 8.4a, above). The bile duct and portal vein are not always parallel along their entire course. Therefore, gun signs may only appear with a certain direction and level of section. There is a nodular formation in contact with the distal segment of the bile duct (black arrow above) However, it is not immediately possible to affirm its pathologic nature. If we follow the bile duct to the nodule (Fig. 8.4b) we see it abruptly taper before it stops. The tapering, irregular diameter and the image of the duct coming to a stop indicate a pathologic nodule, probably tumoral.

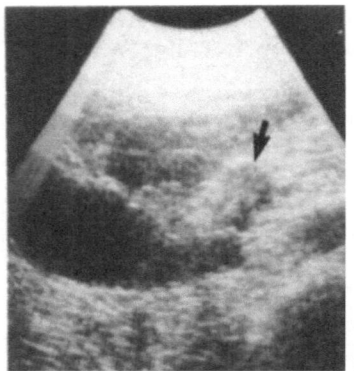 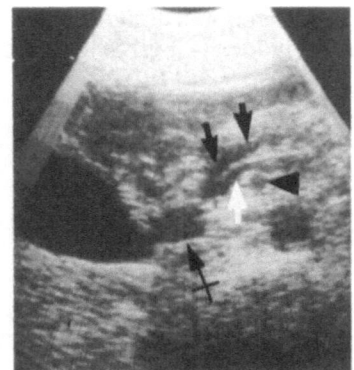

c

d

Fig. 8.4

Its pathologic nature is confirmed by analysis of transverse sections (Fig. 8.4c, above). The echogenicity of the nodule (arrow) contrasts with the adjacent pancreatic tissue.

Now the pancreatic duct:

In Fig. 8.4d you immediately noticed a distinct dilatation of the pancreatic duct (black arrows, above). It is clearly the pancreatic duct since it runs anterior to the splenic vein (white arrow), which is itself identified by the section of the superior mesenteric artery (arrowhead).
The oval element found between the ductal elements (pancreatic duct and splenic vein), on the one hand, and the gall bladder on the other corresponds to the transverse section of the dilated common bile duct (‡).

Thus we have confirmed the binomial sign and discovered the lesion responsible for it, which corresponds to a small ampulloma.

Are additional procedures necessary?

The tumoral nature of the nodule cannot be immediately confirmed. Guided puncture would be needed for this purpose but there is no point in this case of jaundice since surgery is required anyway. CT is useful once a tumor has been demonstrated, in order to specify its local extension. Instrumental cholangiography is not justified in such a case.

8.5. Mr. Chestnut has a chronic disease likely to cause non-obstructive jaundice. When his complexion turns yellow, friends, relatives, and physician begin to throw up their hands, expecting the worst. But since there is a discrepancy with the biological tests, the patient is referred for a sonographic examination.

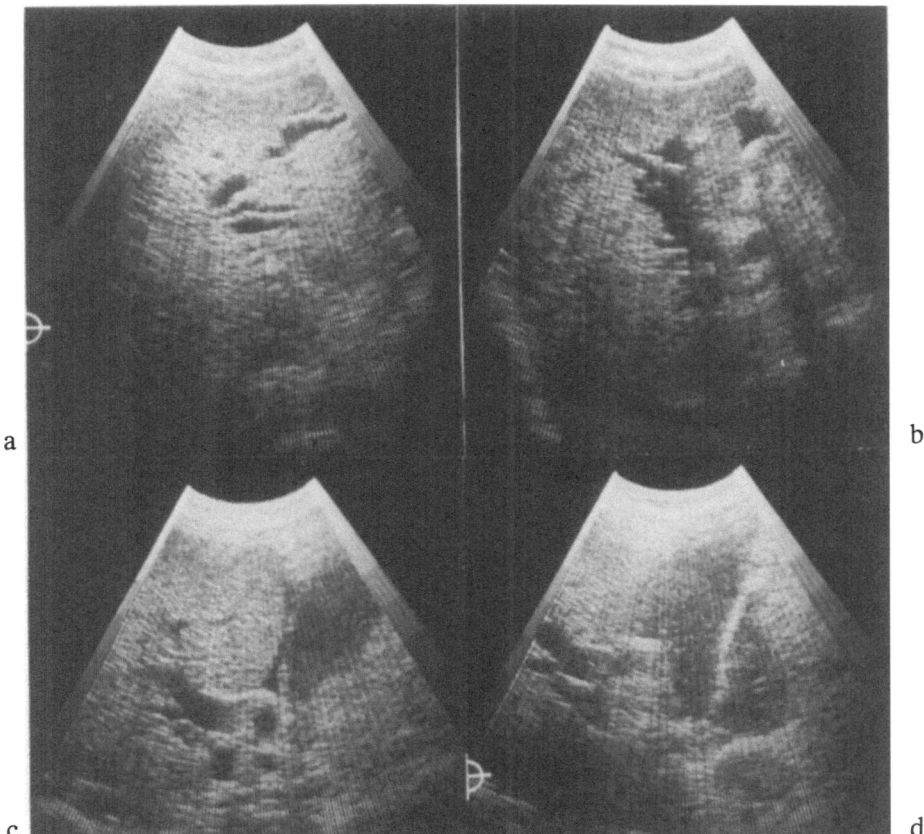

Fig. 8.5. a Transverse section, **b** intercostal section, **c, d** sagittal sections

a) Are there objective signs of dilatation?

Yes, certainly, and in every section. Transverse section 8.5a (below) shows several intrahepatic gun signs (arrows).

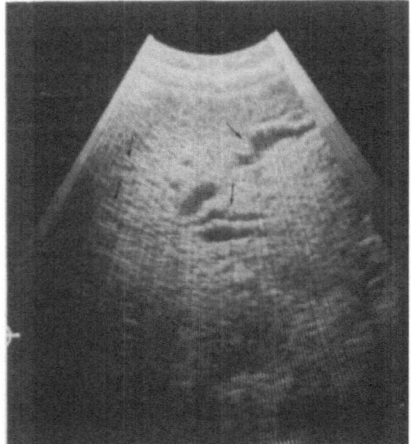

Fig. 8.5a

Intercostal section 8.5b shows a very large right branch of the hepatic duct (↓).

The parallel portal branch, not seen here, can be identified in real time by its relation to the portal vein. But you have analysed another relevant feature in the scan...

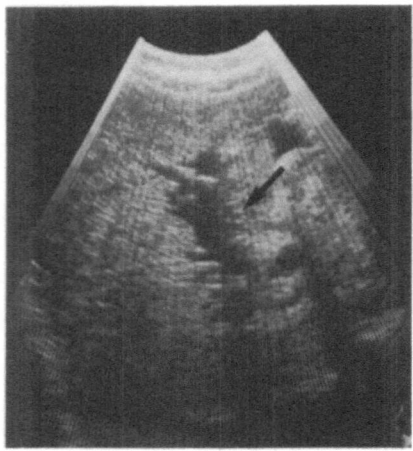

Fig. 8.5b

...It is the good sound transmission of the duct's contents, characterised by a posterior echo amplitude enhancement. This is due to the high protein concentration of bile, leading to a lower attenuation than in blood (Cosgrove).

Parallel sagittal sections show a subhepatic gun sign at the level of the common bile duct (black arrow, Fig. 8.5c, d, below). You have noticed some sludge in the gall bladder infundibulum (white arrow). Gall bladder sludge and gun sign confirm the diagnosis of obstruction.

c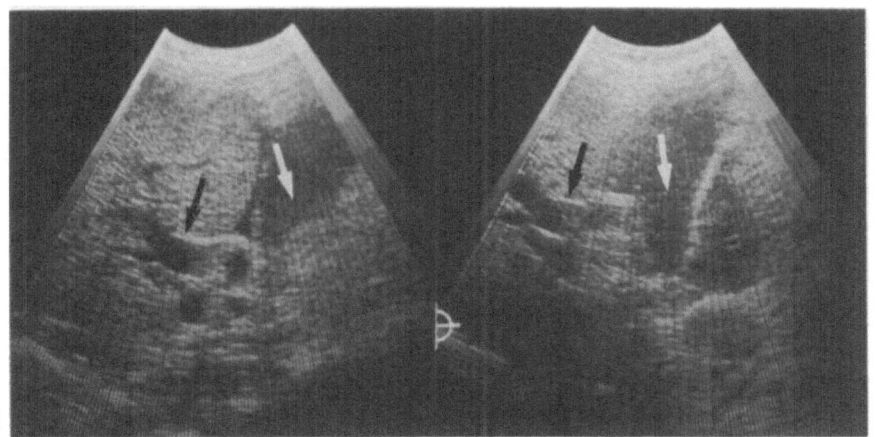d

Fig. 8.5

b) What is the level of the obstruction?

The subhepatic gun sign indicates that the obstruction is low.

c) What is its nature?

Parasagittal section 8.5d shows a pancreatic tumoral nodule (white arrow, below).

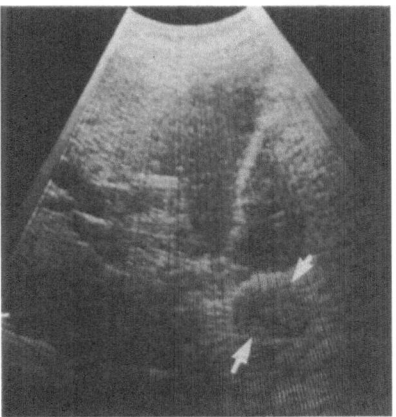

Fig. 8.5d

d) Finally, what was the chronic, potentially icterogenic disease the patient was suffering from at the beginning?

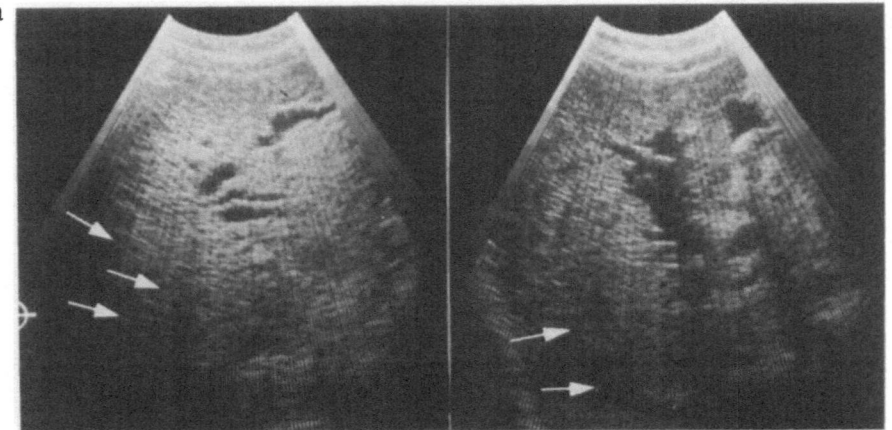

Fig. 8.5

Sections 8.5a and b through the liver show an accentuated attenuation with depth (arrows, above).

More importantly, ascites is visible between the liver and gall bladder in section 8.5c below (arrows), as well as below the gall bladder in section 8.5d (arrow). Now look once again at Fig. 8.5c. Where do you locate the small fluid collections visualized posterior to the portal vein? (Answer[1] at bottom of page.)

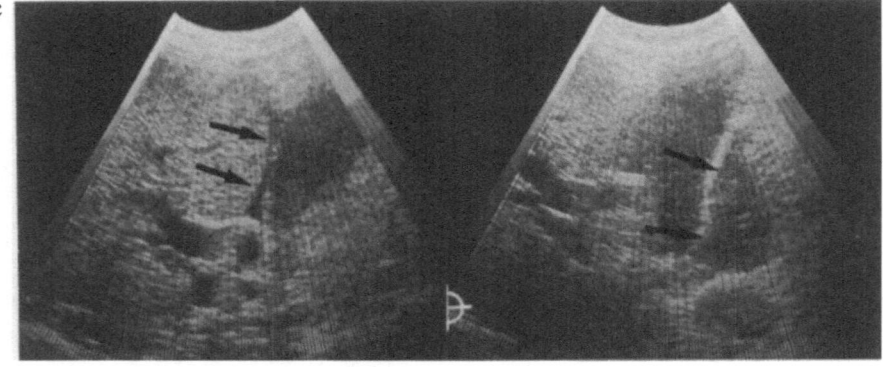

Fig. 8.5

This ascites may be due to the peritoneal extension of the pancreatic carcinoma. This should be verified by a cytological study. But clearly the patient has cirrhosis; in any case the disease was previously diagnosed and followed up. Should other procedures be carried out?
CT is advisable for better knowledge of the tumoral extension.
Should guided puncture be carried out to confirm the malignant nature of the pancreatic nodule? In fact, a biliary by-pass will be performed in this patient; surgical biopsy can be carried out then. In any case, whatever the histological nature of the mass, a duodenopancreatectomy is certainly not called for in the light of this cirrhotic patient's frail condition and underlying poor prognosis.

---

1 in Winslow's foramen

8.6. Mrs. Pecan is not yellow, but comparison of her ultrasound documents with the previous patient's may be interesting.

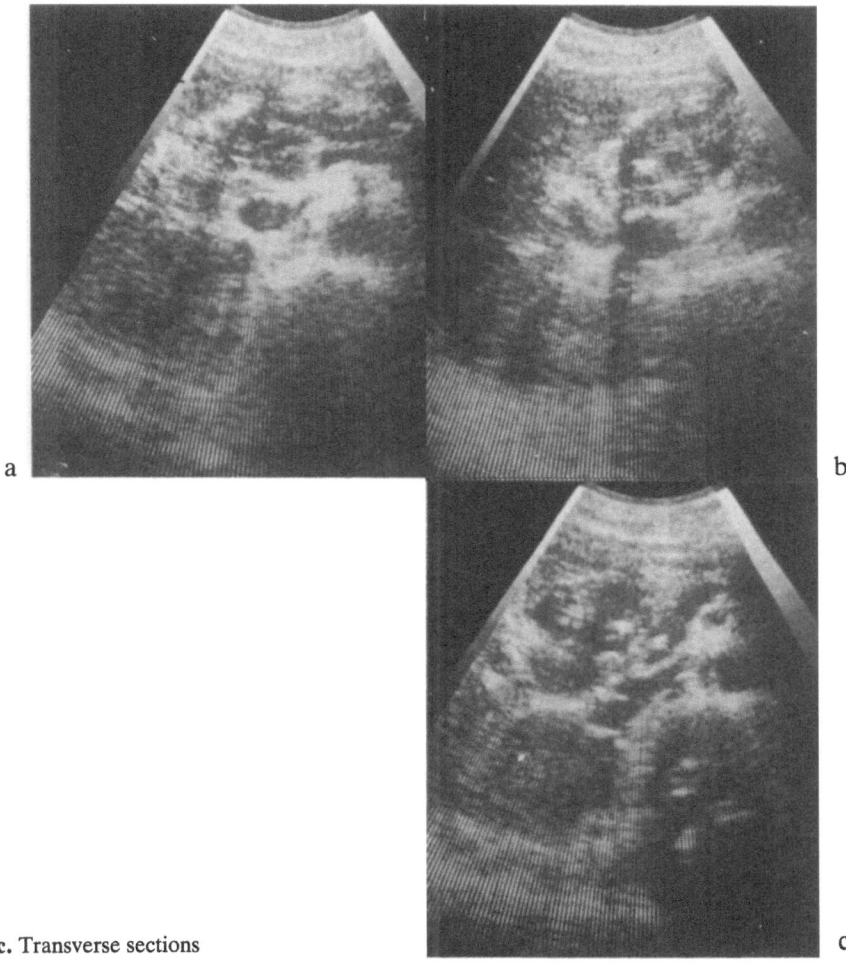

Fig. 8.6a–c. Transverse sections

What do you think of the pancreas in Fig. 8.6a?

The pancreas is enlarged, heterogeneous (arrows, Fig. 8.6a, below) and above all...

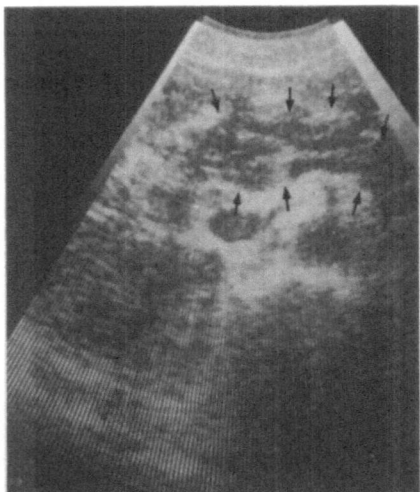

Fig. 8.6a

...it contains a dilated pancreatic duct.

The linear sonotransparency of the pancreatic duct (arrows, below) is clearly delineated within the pancreatic tissue, anterior to the splenic vein (↓ V, below).

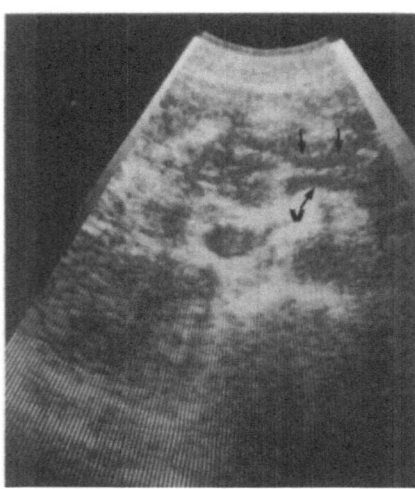

Fig. 8.6a

More caudal parallel sections (Fig. 8.6b, c, below) show a large swelling of the pancreatic head. Its echotexture is heterogeneous and multinodular (↓).

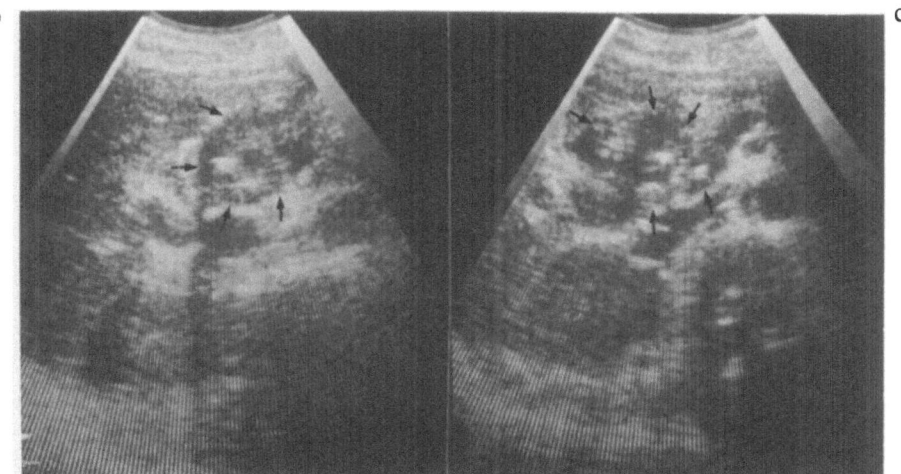

Fig. 8.6

The echostructure is very different from that of the pancreatic tumors already observed (Figs. 1.1, 8.5d). They were less heterogeneous and more sonolucent. Images such as those of Fig. 8.6 are strongly suggestive of chronic pancreatitis. In 60% of chronic pancreatitis cases the dilated pancreatic duct has a zigzag course which is missing here. (Zipper-like pancreatic duct.)

What does the shadow (arrow, Fig. 8.6b, below) correspond to?

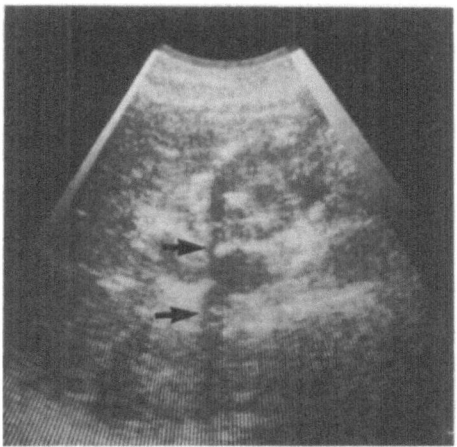

Fig. 8.6b

It is due to sound refraction and does not indicate the presence of air or calcium.

103

8.7. We would now like you to give your opinion of the pancreatic swelling in Mr. Palmetto who, like the previous patient, is not yellow.

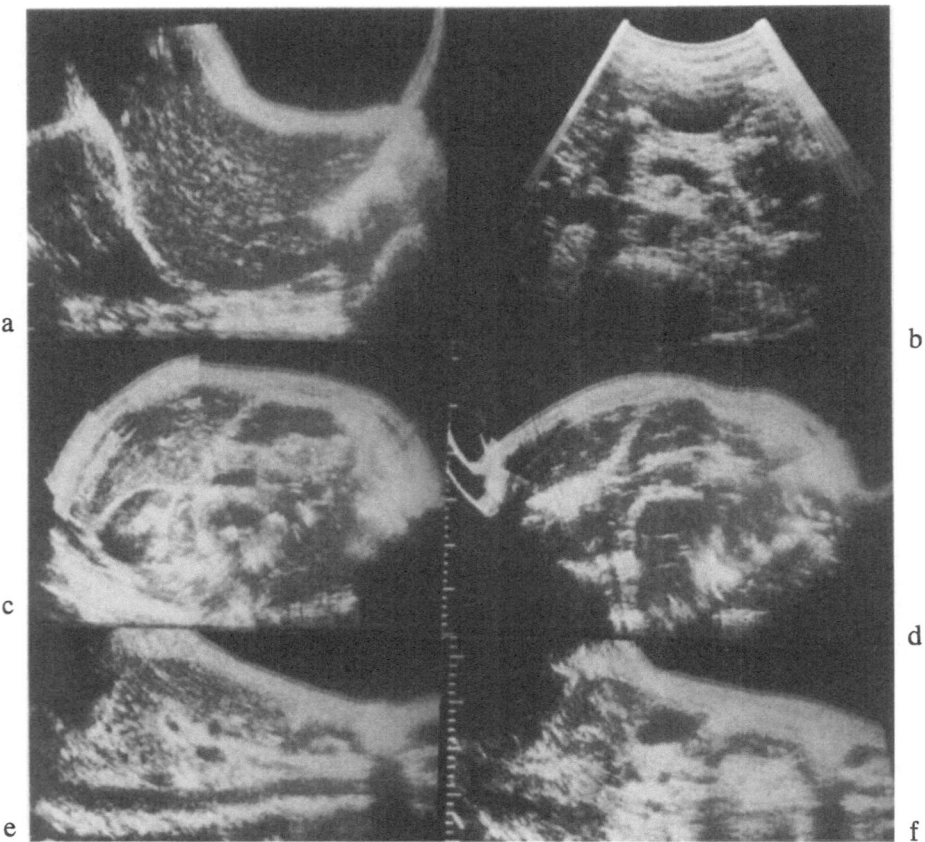

Fig. 8.7.a, e, f Sagittal sections, **b–d** transverse sections

The mass shown in Fig. 8.7c, d (arrows, below) is sonolucent. So it is a...

c̃
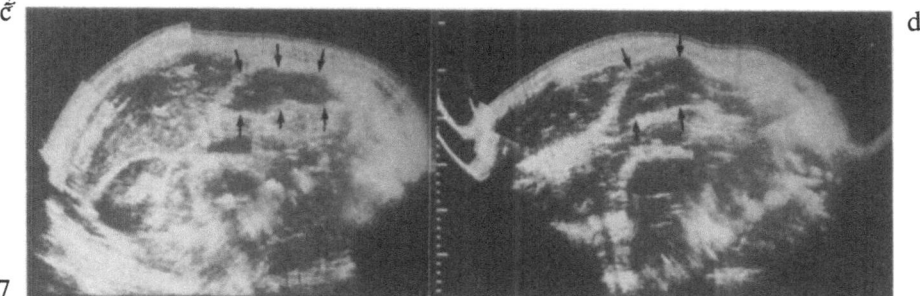
d

Fig. 8.7

... It is a pancreatic carcinoma.
But be careful! Subcutaneous inflammations superimposed on chronic pancreatitis result in similar images; hence the importance of guided puncture. In fact transverse section 8.7b showed you that the pancreas *(P)* was normal despite compression of its body by an adjacent mass (arrows, below).

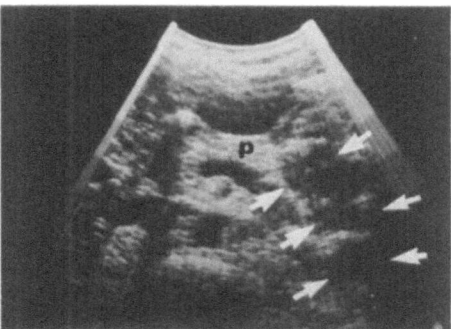
Fig. 8.7b

If the scans showed only this mass, it might correspond to a pancreatic cancer arising from the anterior aspect of the gland. Actually, sections 8.7b–d show multiple nodular elements whose multiplicity indicate their ganglionic nature. This is clearly apparent in Fig. 8.7b (above): at least three nodules (arrows) can be seen anterior to the left kidney. You have also noticed a normal digestive-tract bull's-eye pattern in front of the most anterior nodules. This is the large bowel, since the fluid-filled stomach is seen anterior to the pancreas.
These multiple prerenal ganglionic nodules also appear in the parallel sections 8.7c, d (arrows, next page). So we are dealing with lymphnodes and not with a pancreatic mass.

The first adenopathies we studied in Figs. 8.7c and d are anterior to the mesenteric vessels and are therefore mesenteric adenopathies.

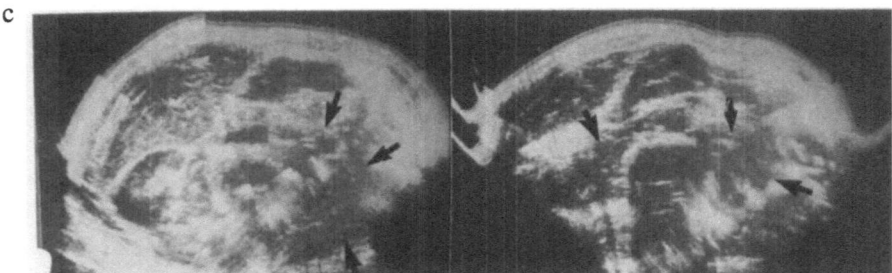

Fig. 8.7

So there are both retroperitoneal and mesenteric adenopathies.

You have discovered another abnormality. There is also (Fig. 8.7a, below) a pleural effusion (↓).

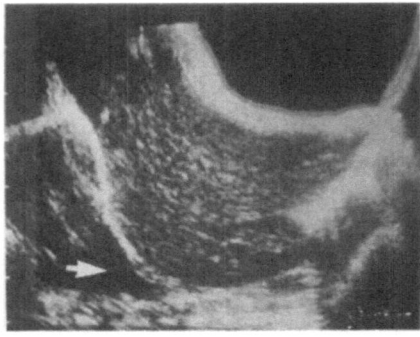

Fig. 8.7a

All these abnormalities, which are consistent with a lymphoma, are actually related to metastases of an embryonic testicular carcinoma.
Besides a chest X-ray, should other procedures be considered for this patient? Lymphography would not give us further relevant information, but CT may aid in the evaluation of the lesions. In some clinically occult testicular tumors, testicular ultrasound can be instrumental in the diagnosis.

Chapter 9

Several Acute Situations

9.1. Mr. Sequoia is 30. Just to get things rolling after that morning coffee, he indulges in a little white wine. After an hour at the wheel of his truck, his throat is dry from all the dust of the road; what's to be done, but wash those tonsils with the help of a few beers...

At 11 o'clock his vision is getting a little blurred, so he refocuses with a little whisky, and so it goes...

One day, this fine, ordinary citizen is hospitalized owing to a violent and painful epigastric attack.

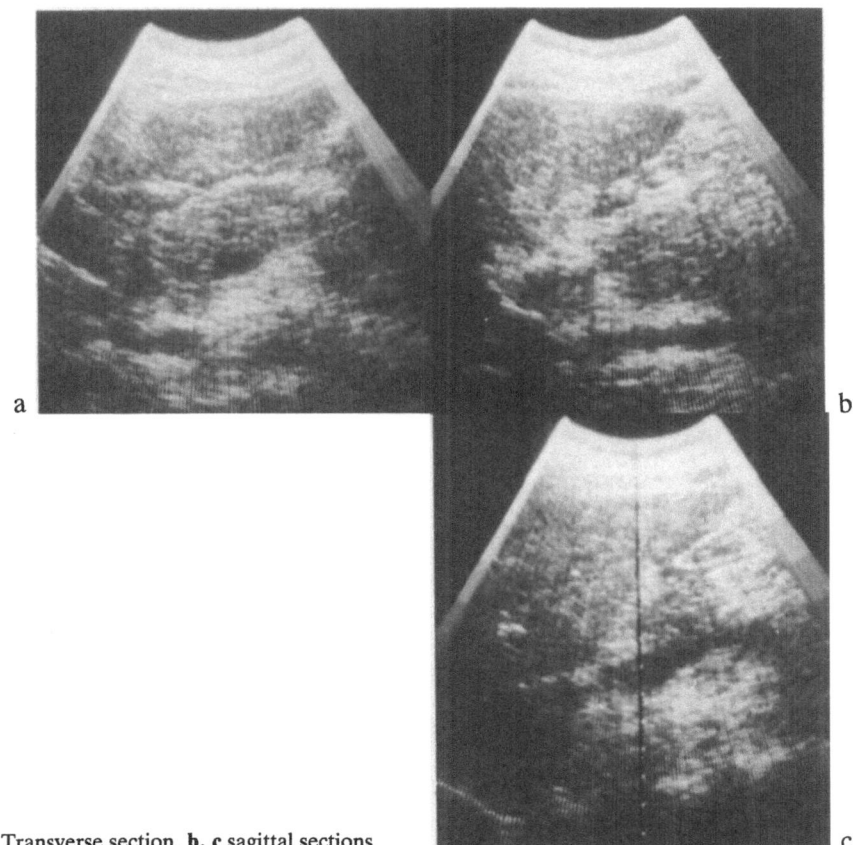

Fig. 9.1. a Transverse section, **b, c** sagittal sections

The pancreas?

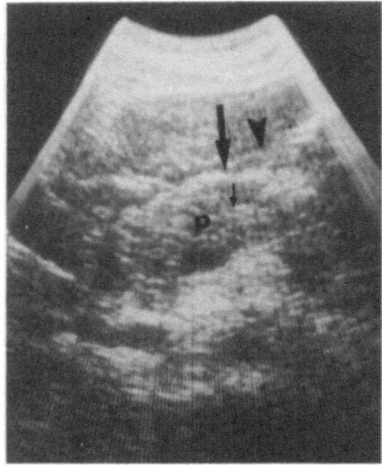

Fig. 9.1a

...It appears abnormaly large (Fig. 9.1a, above), particularly at the level of the neck (↓, *p*).

The pancreatic duct (small arrow, above), whose linear reflexion appears anterior to the space separating the mesenteric vein from the adjacent artery, is not enlarged. The reflectivity of the pancreas is identical to that of the liver: therefore, it is slightly diminished. The elongated bull's-eye pattern of the stomach (arrowhead, above) is seen posterior to the liver and anterior to the echogenic pancreatic fat. Now look at sagittal sections 9.1b, c below. The pancreatic swelling (↓) is seen anterior to the vena cava *(c)* and around the mesenteric vein *(V)*.

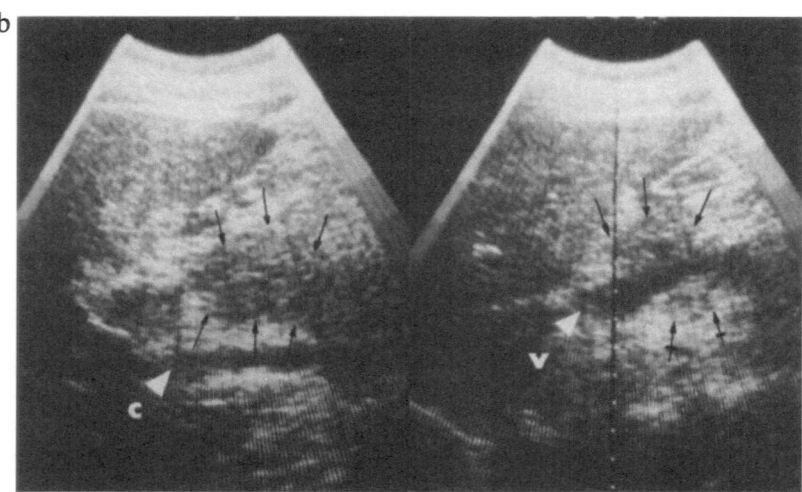

Fig. 9.1

The prevenous pancreatic tissue (↓) is cephalic. The retrovenous glandular tissue (crossed arrow) belongs to the uncinate process.

The pain and the appearance of the pancreas allow us to conclude that this is acute pancreatitis.

We re-examine the patient 24 hours later (Fig. 9.1d, e, below). The pancreatic image is little changed. You should however notice an apparently new feature...

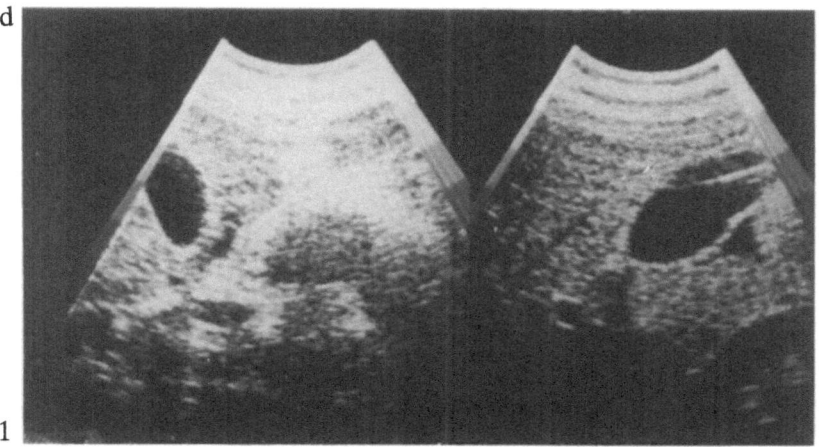

d   e

Fig. 9.1

If you haven't identified it, look at Fig. 9.1e below.

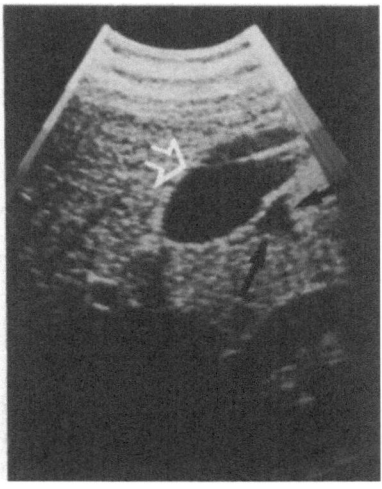

Fig. 9.1e

It's a sagittal section through the gall bladder (open arrow) and right kidney. This section shows a sonotransparent triangle (black arrows) adjacent to the posterior wall of the gall bladder. Thus, there is fluid in the peritoneal cavity.

109

If we look again at Fig. 9.1d (p. 109, then below), we also find a fluid strip (↓) between the gall bladder (open arrow) and the descending portion of the duodenum, near the pancreas *(P)*. It is in the right part of the lesser sac, at the level of the aditus.

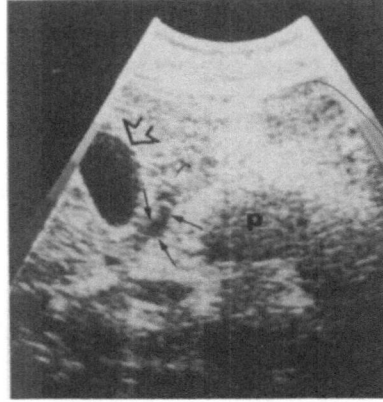

Fig. 9.1d

Look again at Fig. 9.1a (p. 107, then below): we find the same fluid image (↓) in the same area; it passed unnoticed.

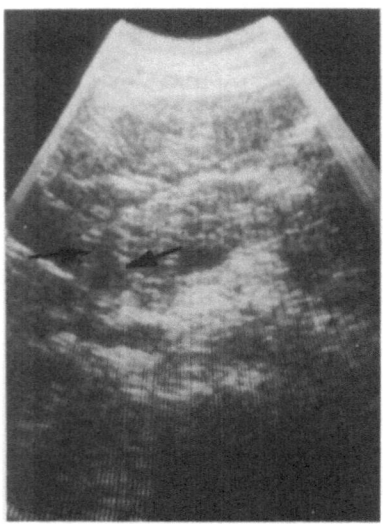

Fig. 9.1a

The presence of intraperitoneal liquid during acute pancreatitis is obviously an important finding. It requires close follow-up to detect necrosis. Curiously enough, while contact of the pancreas with the peritoneal cavity is essentially by way of the lesser omental sac, fluid is not always encountered here. This is probably due to the dynamic phenomena described by Morton Meyers[1].

1 Dynamic Radiology of the Abdomen, 1977, Springer-Verlag, Heidelberg New York

Can we locate the lesser omental sac in these sections? Of course, since the stomach (Fig. 9.1a–c) is clearly seen anterior to the pancreas. It is characterized by the linear sonotransparency of its wall (arrows below).

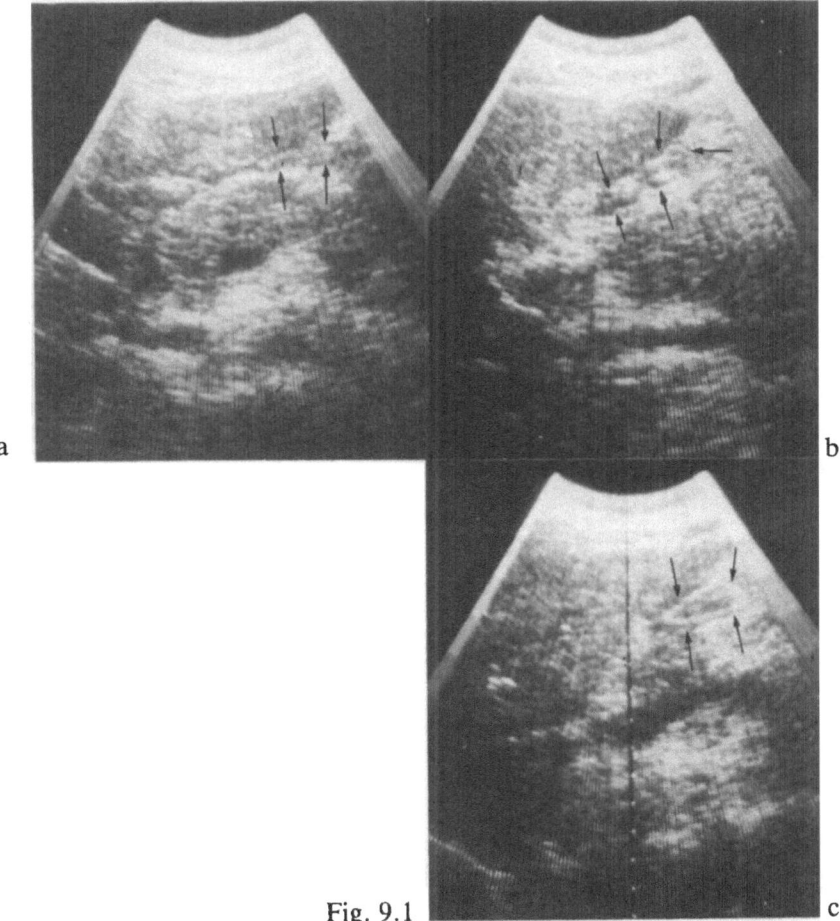

Fig. 9.1

The lesser sac, which is virtual at this level, is found between the gland and posterior gastric wall.

Should other procedures be carried out? If the reduction in swelling is not rapid, or if the initial swelling is great, contrast CT is essential: prenecrotic pancreatic tissue does not blush. An excellent map of the pancreas will be obtained, allowing differentiation of peri-pancreatic edema from pancreatic tissue, and of normal pancreatic tissue from tissue threatened by necrosis. Unless the necrotic cavity is distinct, the ultrasound image of diffuse swelling is unspecific.

9.2. Mr. Mulberry's clinical history is similar to Mr. Sequoia's.

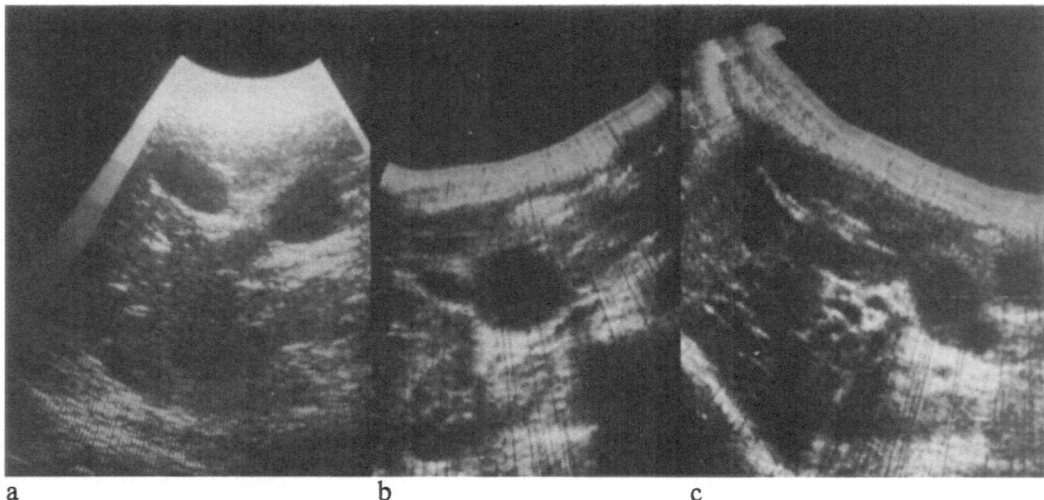

a   b   c

Fig. 9.2. a, b Transverse sections, **c** sagittal section

What does transverse section 9.2a show?

... It shows the fluid collection of a pseudocyst (arrows, below) indicating rapid progress of pancreatic necrosis.

The other image of a more external fluid collection obviously belongs to the gall bladder.

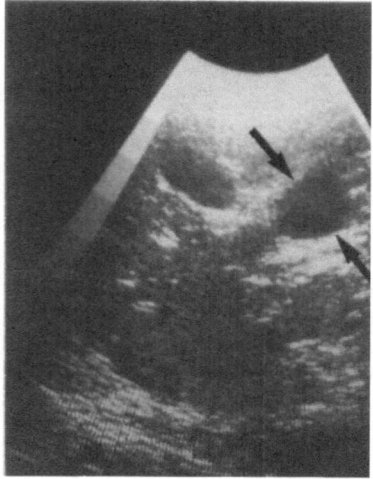

Fig. 9.2a

Twenty-four hours later, we find the same image (Fig. 9.2b, black arrow, below) with a sediment of small necrotic debris (white arrows).

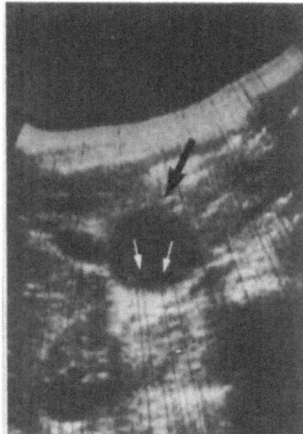

Fig. 9.2b

Sagittal section 9.2c (p. 112, then below) reveals three cavities (↓) in an enormous cephalic swelling (open arrows). There is no intraperitoneal fluid.

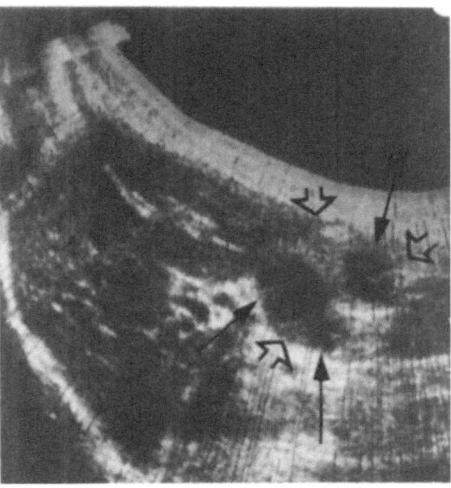

Fig. 9.2c

The patient leaves refusing both surgery and drainage by guided puncture.

Figures 9.2d, e are sections taken 4 months later. What differences do you see in comparison with the previous sections?

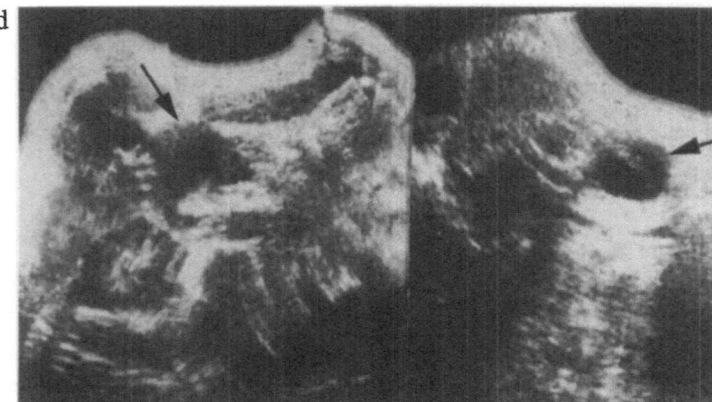

Fig. 9.2

There is now only one cavity (↓) and a very thick wall has formed: the pseudocyst is mature.

Should additional procedures be carried out?

Certainly not when the pseudocyst is mature unless there are symptoms of portal hypertension or biliary dilatation.
However, during the acute period of pancreatic necrosis, CT will show diffusion of the edema, or fluid migration, where deep suppuration may eventually develop. As a rule, these fluid migrations (mediastinal, intraperitoneal, retroperitoneal) are shown by sonography. Sonography is however sometimes unsuccessful in certain areas of the lower abdomen.

After necrosis, should an arteriography be systematically carried out to detect false aneurysms caused by maturation of the arterial wall?

This is still an open question. Contrast CT will detect some of these lesions. The Danish School (Holm) punctures developing pseudocysts. This puncture may relieve pain and aid in the regression of the pseudocysts, which may also regress spontaneously. Puncture also makes possible the injection of a contrast medium to detect communication with the pancreatic ductal network; this policy is not universally accepted.

Now look at Fig. 9.2f, below.

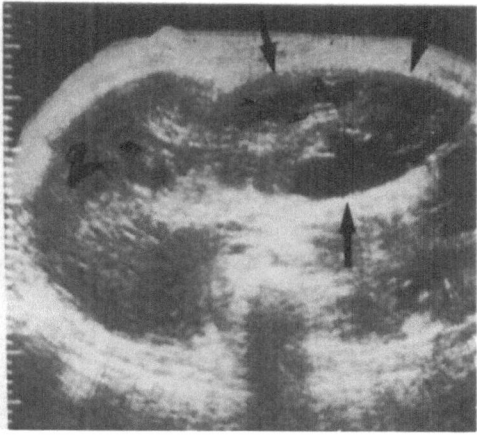

Fig. 9.2f

This scan performed at the end of a painful attack, shows a subcapsular fluid collection (↓) at the level of the left hepatic lobe. This fluid is of pancreatic origin and due to acute pancreatitis. We reprint this scan[1] for two reasons:

a) To remind you that during acute pancreatitis pancreatic juice may spread anywhere.

b) To give you a chance to check if you remember the origins of such subcapsular hepatic collections, namely:
   - Abscess
   - Biliary collections (biloma)
   - Traumatic hematomas (following puncture or surgery), or spontaneous hematomas (due to impaired blood coagulation or tumoral hemorrhage)
   - Collections of pancreatic origin

1 From "Ultrasonography of Digestive Diseases", Mosby Publ., St. Louis, USA, 1982

9.3. Mr. Oak is admitted after a severe collapse accompanied by sharp pain in the right upper quadrant.

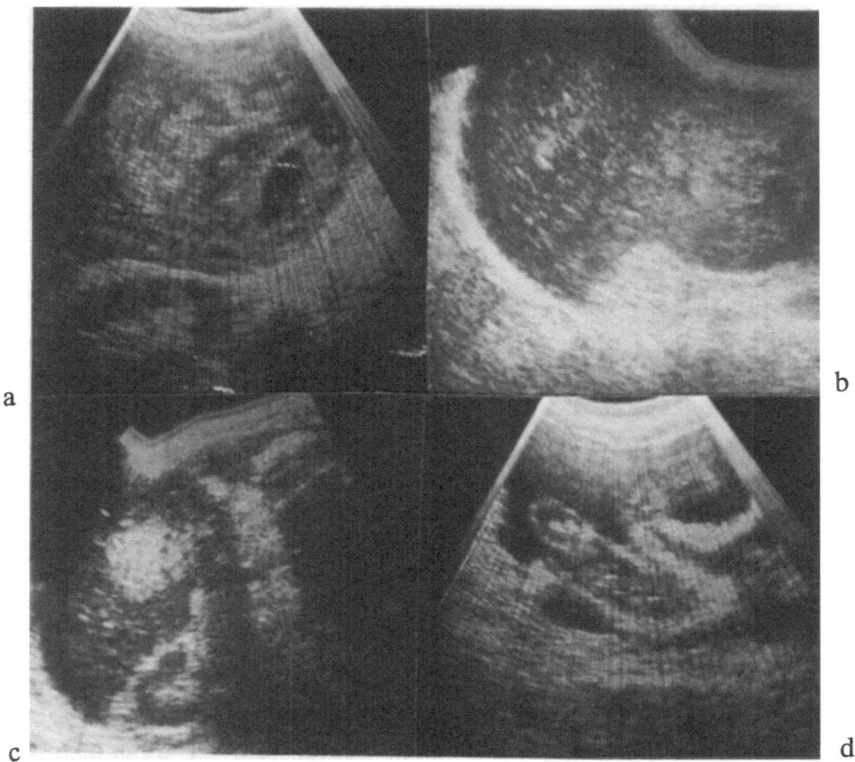

Fig. 9.3. a, b Sagittal sections, **c** transverse section, **d** right coronal section

Sagittal section 9.3a shows a tumoral liver: a large necrotic lesion (↓ below) distends the infrarenal hump.

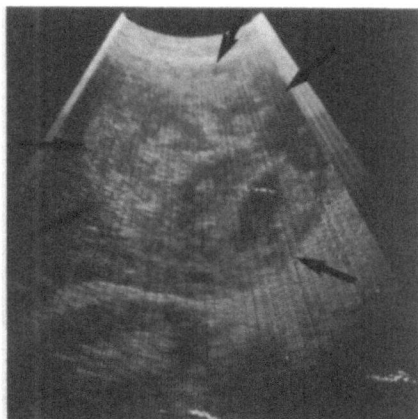

Fig. 9.3a

What else have you noticed?

You have seen a very narrow sonotransparent strip (↓ below) between the liver and perirenal fat. This is a "crescent moon" sign, indicating the presence of fluid in Morison's pouch.

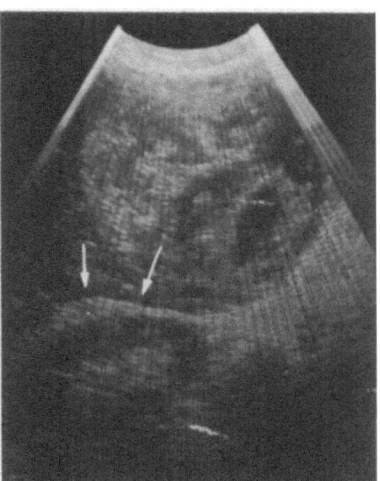

Fig. 9.3a

Figure 9.3e (below) shows a crescent moon sign (↓) in another patient.

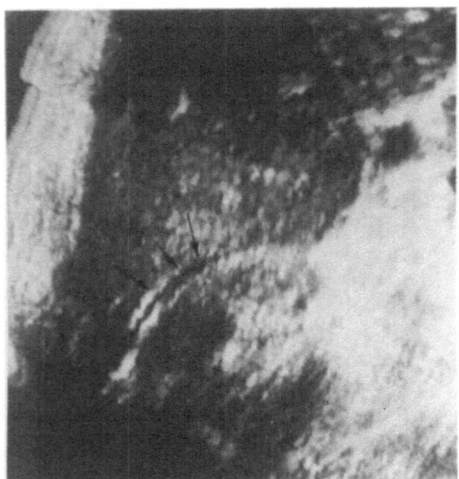

Fig. 9.3e

What else have you seen in this section?

... There are multiple hepatic nodules of metastatic origin (white arrows, below).

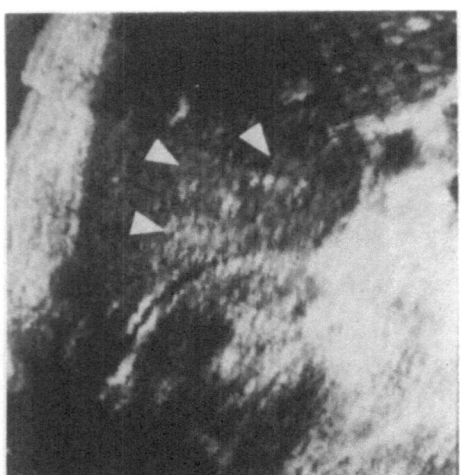

Fig. 9.3e

Let's get back to Mr. Oak. There's a large quantity of intraperitoneal fluid (↓ Fig. 9.3b, c, d, p. 116, then below).

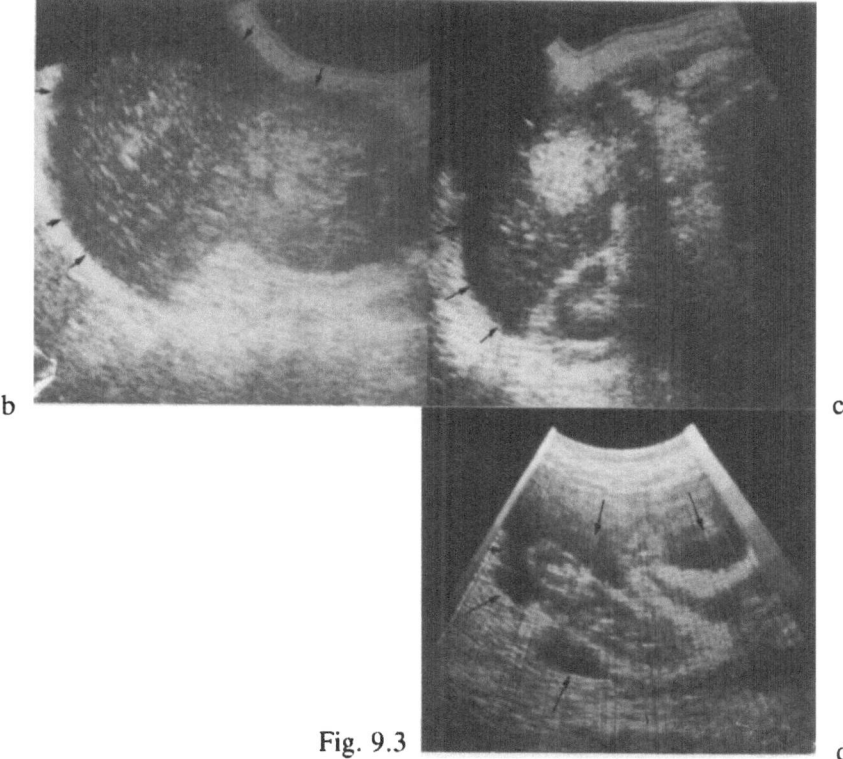

Fig. 9.3

Fluid surrounds the tumoral liver; intestinal loops float within the effusion (Fig. 9.3d, above: ↓ = peri-intestinal fluid). The association of a tumoral liver, collapse, and intraperitoneal fluid should make us think of hemoperitoneum, caused by hemorrhage from a hypervascularized hepatoma. Abdominal puncture will immediately confirm the hemoperitoneum.

What should the next procedure be?

Arteriography, as the first step in embolization.

9.4. Miss Sumac is 15. She complains of sharp pelvic pains. She is very pale and her pulse is accelerated.

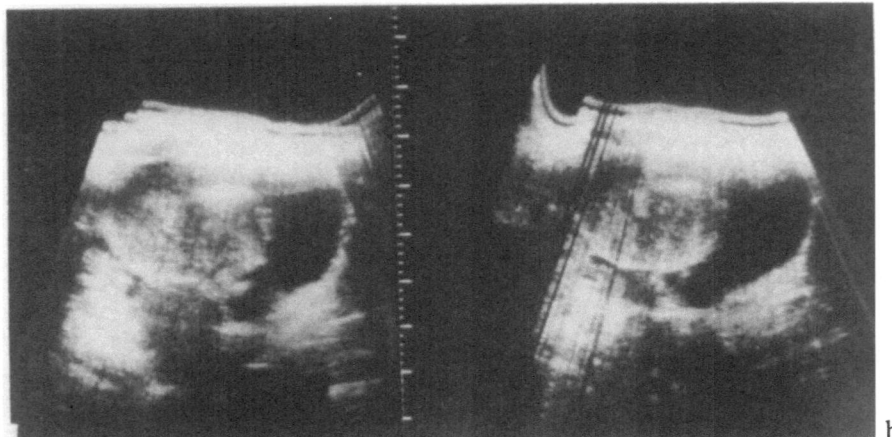

a   b

Fig. 9.4a, b. Transverse sections

The pelvic sections show a fluid collection (black arrows) above the bladder (open arrow).

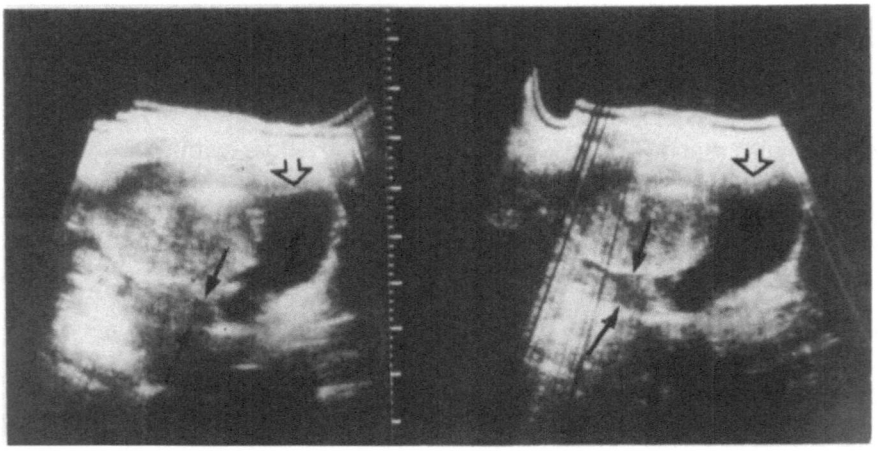

a   b

Fig. 9.4

The uterus is very large (open arrows) and surrounded by fluid. The first hypothesis is hemoperitoneum caused by a ruptured tubal pregnancy.
But the relevant clinical history is lacking. The patient denies previous sexual intercourse, moreover, the "uterus" is too large.

a 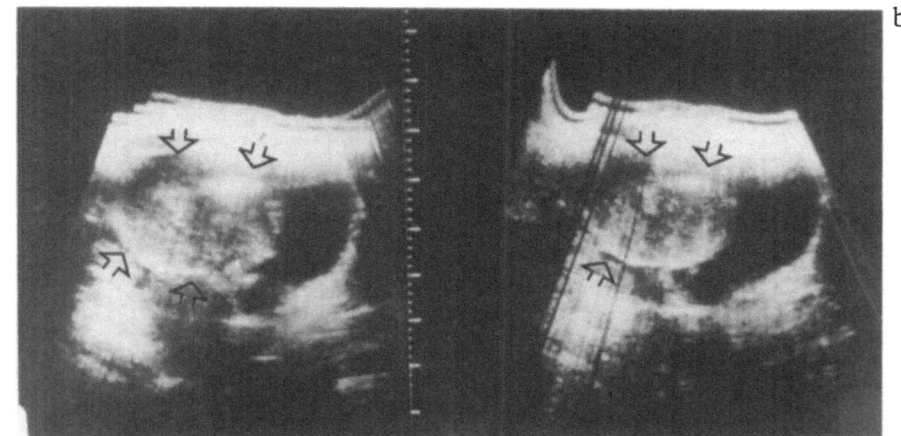 b

Fig. 9.4

But we don't waste too much time thinking: the situation is acute. The patient is operated on. The fluid is not hemorrhagic; there is only a slightly tinted serosity. The uterus is normal. The round pelvic mass is not the uterus but a prolapsed and twisted intestinal loop in Douglas' pouch.

Moral:

a) Always carry out a detailed anatomical analysis. The normal uterus should have been identified in this pelvis, which was well contrasted owing to intraperitoneal fluid. The sonologist jumped too quickly to false anatomic conclusions, confirming a gynecological process, more or less suggested by clinical history. Clinical data are indispensable during radiological procedures, but one must keep an open mind to make an accurate interpretation of the images.
b) In emergency cases, sonography will often confirm the urgency (intraperitoneal effusion) and indicate the abnormal zone with greater precision than mere palpation. But it does not always result in an accurate diagnosis. One must know one's limits, as Socrates used to say whenever he began an ultrasound examination: γνῶθι σεαυτόν.

121

9.5. Mrs. Blackgum complains of abdominal pains and distension. The situation is becoming acute. The left lumbar fossa is tender.

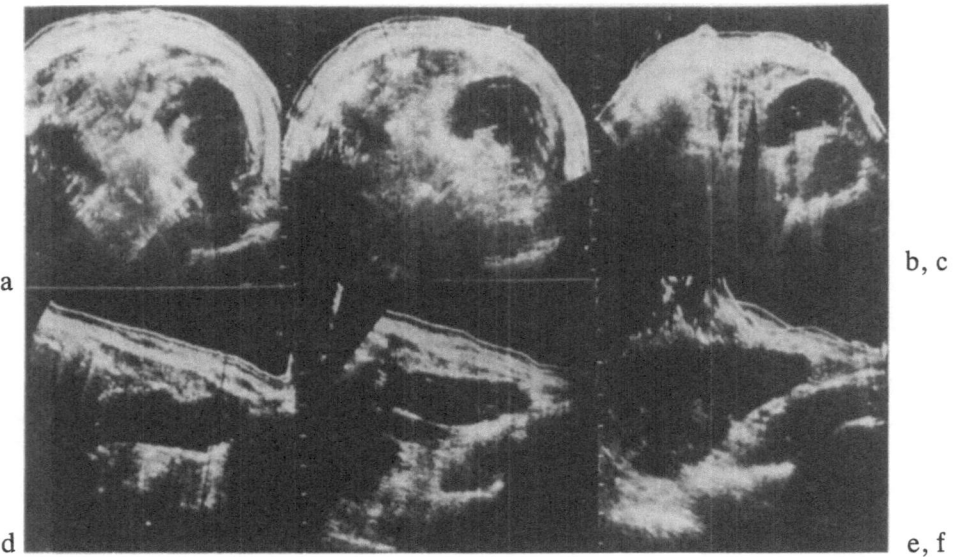

a   b, c

d   e, f

Fig. 9.5. a–c Transverse sections, **d–f** sagittal sections

After studying Fig. 9.5 there's a question you should ask the patient (or her physician). What question?

... "Are you receiving (is she receiving) anticoagulant therapy?"

There is a large deep collection (↓ below, Fig. 9.5a–c): For a cardiac patient taking anticoagulants, the diagnosis of the collection is obvious: hematoma.

Where is it located?

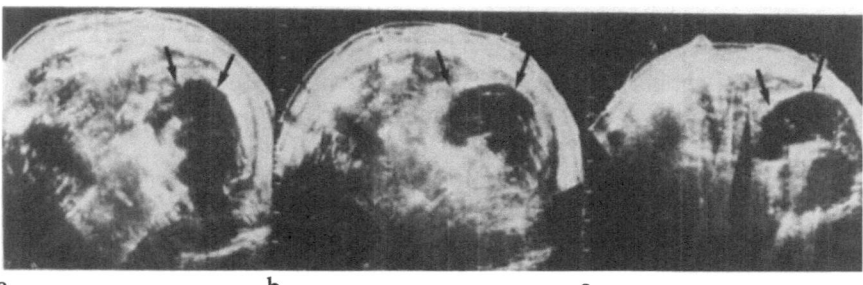

a   b   c

Fig. 9.5

122

Now's the time to look at parasagittal sections 9.5df (below).

Fig. 9.5

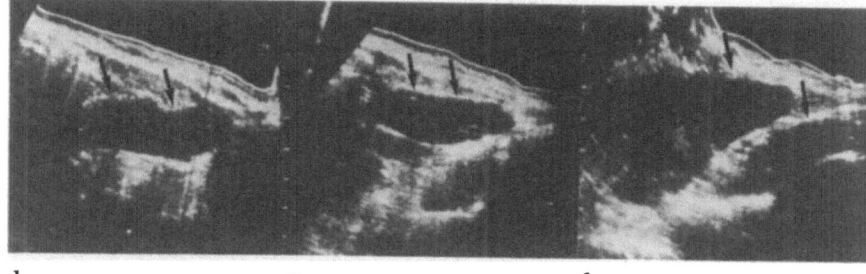

d   e   f

The elongated shape of the collection (↓) does not favor a hematoma of the intestinal wall. It clearly is not a hematoma of the anterior abdominal wall, nor a hemoperitoneum. It's a retroperitoneal hematoma. If you look at Fig. 9.5e, f, you will in fact see two adjacent collections (arrows below) with the same orientation. How do you explain them?

The explanation is anatomical; it is made easier by Fig. 9.5c, p. 122 and below.

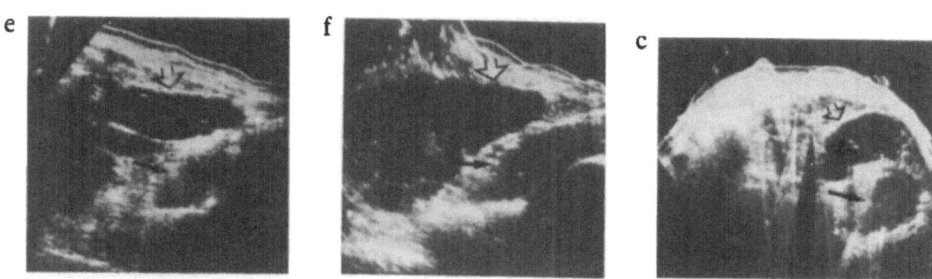

e   f   c

Fig. 9.5

The deeper collection (arrow) is a hematoma of the psoas sheath. The more anterior collection (open arrow) is located in the lower pararenal space. The slight difference in reflectiveness of these two collections may be due to their difference in age; it may also be due to the echogenicity of the muscle itself.
Mrs. Blackgum was operated on. The volume of each hematoma was greater than one liter. It would be illusory to hope for spontaneous reabsorption of such hematomas. It would also be illusory to hope to drain such a hematoma by guided drainage. Absence of a direct approach and the presence of clots call for surgical intervention. Complete evacuation is absolutely necessary, otherwise retroperitoneal fibrosis, liable to induce nervous complications, may develop.

Conclusions

It is of course rather artificial to analyse a few selected scans when the sonologist, who carries out a radiological and clinical examination, sees a considerable number of different images, particularly in real time.

Practice in thorough analysis of associated or successive patterns is, however, fundamental for learning to interpret correctly, and even to carry out an ultrasound examination. With such a training, one will succeed in applying a rigorous, systematic technique to continuous variations, in a process of action and reaction, according to immediate morphological observations and clinical data.

In this field, as in all other fields of morphological diagnosis, Antoine Béclère's maxim remains fundamental: one sees only what one looks for; one looks only for that which one knows.

We also hope to have shown you, in these few examples, how useful it can be to combine sonography with other diagnostic modalities. But also, how easy it is to economize on other procedures, thanks to ultrasound screening, each diagnostic step being part of a logical policy.

The success of a rational methodology, essentially founded on the real time technique, should not cause one to forget the inherent limits of all diagnostic methods, as well as the risk of human error. There comes a time when one should know to stop constructing diagnostic hypotheses and begin discussing treatment, rather than developing false diagnoses.

S. N. Hassani
Real Time Ophthalmic Ultrasonography
In collaboration with R. L. Bard
1978. 423 figures. XXI, 214 pages. ISBN 3-540-90318-6

S. N. Hassani
Ultrasonography of the Abdomen
With a contribution by R. L. Bard
1976. 215 figures. XVI, 127 pages. ISBN 3-540-90166-3

S. N. Hassani
Ultrasound in Gynecology and Obstetrics
In collaboration with R. L. Bard
1978. 337 figures. XX, 182 pages. ISBN 3-540-90260-0

R. O. Meudt, M. Hinselmann
Ultrasonoscopic (real time) Differential Diagnosis in Obstetrics and Gynecology
Echoskopische Differential-Diagnose in Geburtshilfe und Gynäkologie
Sémiologie échoscopique en obstétrique et gynécologie
Semiologia ecoscópica en obstetricia y ginecologia
Semiologia ecoscopica in ostetricia e ginecologia
2nd revised edition. 1978. 209 figures, 1 fold-out table. X, 145 pages. ISBN 3-540-08839-3

Renal Sonography
By F. S. Weill, E. Bihr, P. Rohmer, F. Zeltner
1981. 207 figures. XII, 134 pages. ISBN 3-540-10398-8
Distribution rights for Japan: Igaku Shoin, Tokyo

M. L. Skolnick
Real-time Ultrasound Imaging in the Abdomen
1981. 386 figures. XI, 241 pages. ISBN 3-540-90570-7

F. S. Weill
Ultraschalldiagnostik in der Gastroenterologie
Übersetzt aus dem Französischen von J. Seidel
1981. 559 Abbildungen. X, 542 Seiten. ISBN 3-540-10613-8

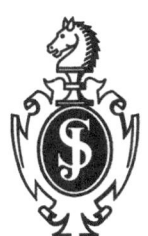

Springer-Verlag
Berlin
Heidelberg
New York
Tokyo

Frontiers in European Radiology

Editors-in-Chief: Albert L. Baert (Leuven), Erik Boijsen (Lund), Walter A. Fuchs (Bern), Friedrich H. W. Heuck (Stuttgart)

Editorial Board: P. Bodart, Brussels; G. Breitling, Tübingen; L. Dalla Palma, Triest; W. Dihlmann, Hamburg; G. du Boulay, London; P. Edholm, Linköping; C. Fauré, Paris; H. Frommhold, Innsbruck; W. Frommhold, Tübingen; T. Greitz, Stockholm; V. Hegedüs, Copenhagen; H. Kauffmann, Berlin; E. Koivisto, Tampere; L. Kreel, London; M. Laval-Jeantet, Paris; A. Lunderquist, Lund; H. J. Middlemiss, Bristol; I. Obrez, Ljubljana; F. Pinet, Lyon; H. Pokieser, Vienna; J. Remy, Lille; P. Rossi, Rome; T. Sherwood, Cambridge; A. Wackenheim, Strasbourg; F. Weill, Besançon

Volume 1
1982. 113 figures in 187 separate illustrations. V, 170 pages
ISBN 3-540-10753-3

Contents: *I. Fernström, B. Johansson:* Percutaneous Extraction of Renal Calculi. – *R. Günther, P. Alken:* Percutaneous Nephropyelostomy and Endo-Urological Manipulations. – *R. Pasariello, G. P. Feltrin, D. Miotto, S. Pedrazzoli, P. Rossi, G. Simonetti:* Transhepatic Portal Catheterization with Pancreatic Venous Sampling Versus Angiography in the Localization of Pancreatic Functioning Tumors. – *G. M. Kauffmann, G. Richter, J. Rassweiler, R. Rohrbach:* New Topics in Embolization. Effects of Central, Peripheral or Capillary Occlusion Type in Animal Models Simulating Tumor Embolization. – *F. Brunelle:* Electric Transcatheter Vascular Obliteration: Electrothrombosis. Electrolysis or Electrocoagulation. – *V. Hegedüs, O. Winding, J. Grønvall, P. Faarup:* Manufacturing-Derived Impurities in Angiography. – *K.-H. Hübener:* Digital Radiography Using a Computed Tomography Instrument.

Volume 2
1982. 70 figures in 84 separate illustrations. V, 103 pages
ISBN 3-540-11349-5

Contents: *W. Loeffler:* NMR as an Imaging Method. – *R. E. Steiner, G. M. Bydder:* Initial Clinical Experience with NMR Imaging. – *F. W. Smith:* NMR Imaging of the Liver and Kidney. – *P. Marhoff, M. Pfeiler:* Digital Fluorography. – *M. P. Capp, S. Nudelman, D. Fisher, T. W. Ovitt, G. D. Pond, M. M. Frost, H. Roehrig, J. Seeger, D. Oimette:* Digital Radiography. – *A. B. Crummy, C. A. Mistretta:* Digital Subtraction Arteriography (DSA). – *T. F. Meaney, M. A. Weinstein, E. Buonocore, J. H. Callagher:* Digital Subtraction Angiography: Cleveland Clinical Experience.

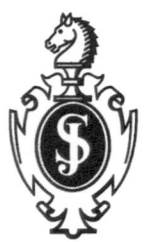

Springer-Verlag
Berlin
Heidelberg
New York
Tokyo